Building
STRONGER BONES
Naturally

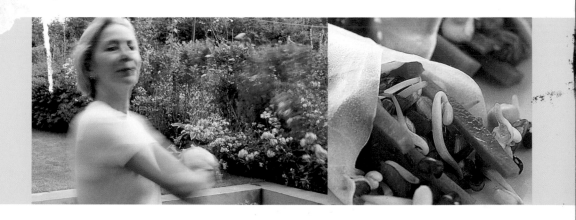

hamlyn

Building
STRONGER BONES
Naturally

Xandria Williams

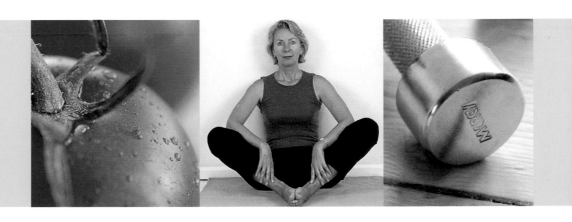

First published in Great Britain in 2002 by Hamlyn,
a division of Octopus Publishing Group Ltd
2–4 Heron Quays, London E14 4JP

ISBN 0 600 60457 8

A CIP catalogue record for this book is available from the
British Library

Printed and bound in China

10 9 8 7 6 5 4 3 2 1

Xandria Williams, MSc, DIC, ARCS, ND, DBM, MRN
Naturopath, Nutritionist, Herbalist, Homeopath, NLP
Practitioner, Personal Development Consultant

Xandria obtained chemistry degrees from Imperial
College, London, then turned to biochemistry and
human metabolism and trained as a naturopath
and nutritionist. She has lectured extensively, both
in undergraduate courses and to graduates and
special interest groups, has written over 350 articles
and 16 books and has appeared frequently on radio
and television.

   She has over twenty years' experience of advising
patients and is currently in private practice in
central London and near Dublin, Ireland.

Xandria can be contacted for consultations in:
London on (44) 020 7824 8153
Ireland on (353) 0405 31191
or alternatively by email to xkw@bigfoot.com

RECIPE NOTES

1. Both metric and imperial measurements have been given in
all recipes. Use one set of measurements only, and not a
mixture of both.
2. Standard level spoon measurements are used in all recipes.
1 tablespoon = one 15 ml spoon
1 teaspoon = one 5 ml spoon
3. Eggs should be large unless otherwise stated. The Department
of Health advises that eggs should not be consumed raw. This
book contains dishes made with raw or lightly cooked eggs.
It is prudent for more vulnerable people such as pregnant and
nursing mothers, invalids, the elderly, babies and young children
to avoid uncooked or lightly cooked dishes made with eggs.
Once prepared, these dishes should be kept refrigerated and
used promptly.
4. Milk should be full fat unless otherwise stated.
5. This book includes dishes made with nuts and nut derivatives.
It is advisable for readers with known allergic reactions to nuts
and nut derivatives and those who may be potentially vulnerable
to these allergies, such as pregnant and nursing mothers,
invalids, the elderly, babies and children to avoid dishes made
with nuts and nut oils. It is also prudent to check the labels
of pre-prepared ingredients for the possible inclusion of nut
derivatives.
6. Pepper should be freshly ground black pepper unless
otherwise stated.
7. Fresh herbs should be used, unless otherwise stated. If
unavailable, use dried herbs as an alternative, but halve the
quantities stated.
8. Ovens should be pre-heated to the specified temperature
– if using a fan-assisted oven, follow the manufacturer's
instructions for adjusting the time and the temperature.
9. Vegetarians should look for the 'V' symbol on a cheese to
ensure it is made with vegetarian rennet. There are vegetarian
forms of Parmesan, feta, Cheddar, Cheshire, Red Leicester,
dolcelatte and many goats' cheeses, among others.

SAFETY NOTE

It is advisable to check with your doctor before embarking on
any exercise or diet programme. *Building Stronger Bones
Naturally* should not be considered a replacement for
professional medical treatment; a physician should be
consulted in all matters relating to health. While the advice and
information in this book is believed to be accurate and the
step-by-step instructions have been devised to avoid strain,
neither the publisher nor the author can accept legal
responsibility for any injury or illness sustained while
following the exercises and advice included.

Contents

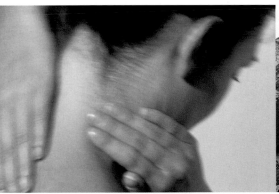
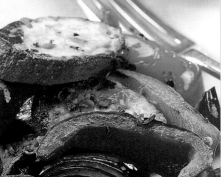

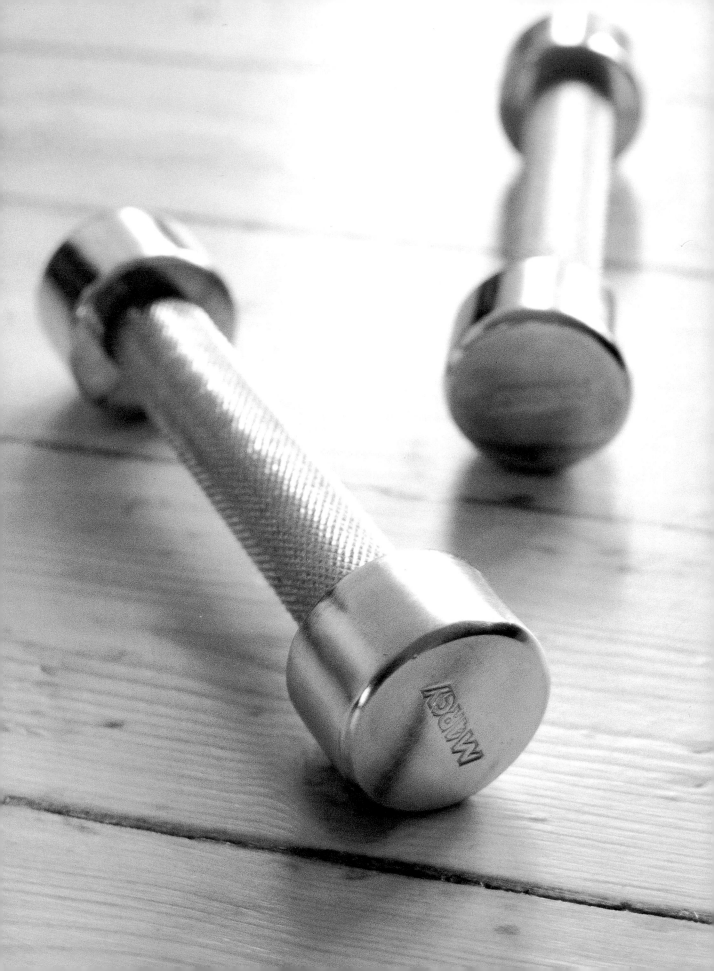

Introduction

The word osteoporosis is linked inextricably in people's minds with the idea of brittle, crumbling bones, and it is widely perceived as being a problem facing older people, especially women. In fact, osteoporosis is only one of several conditions involving faulty bone structure, and it does not mean that your bones are crumbling. It does mean, however, that your bones are becoming more and more fragile and are liable to break with increasing ease.

The incidence of osteoporosis has increased in Western countries in recent years, and this increase seems to be the result of both the food we eat and our lifestyles. People with fragile bones often suffer recurrent or persistent pain and the consequences of broken bones, usually a hip, for elderly people can mean increased isolation and limited mobility. This book shows how you can take positive action, by changing your diet and by making a few changes to your life, to avoid the onset of bone problems later in life.

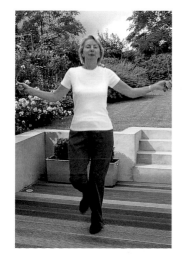

It looks at the nature and structure of bones in some detail, showing how the food we eat affects the way they grow and develop. It assesses what our bones need for maximum health and strength and, on the negative side, what factors have adverse effects on them and the habits and practices that constitute risk factors for the development of osteoporosis. This leads to a more detailed discussion of lifestyle, of diet and the best foods to eat for our bones, of nutritional supplements that can be taken to support the diet and of exercises, ranging from the gentle to the more robust, that can be undertaken to maintain good bone health. The recipes included in Part 3 will show you that there are many simple ways you can change your diet to the benefit of your bones.

Developing and maintaining healthy bones that will last all life long may not seem to be a priority, but this hidden problem will affect an increasing number of us, and if we are to remain active and independent as we grow older it is important to take steps now and to make the changes in our lives that will improve our quality of life in the long term.

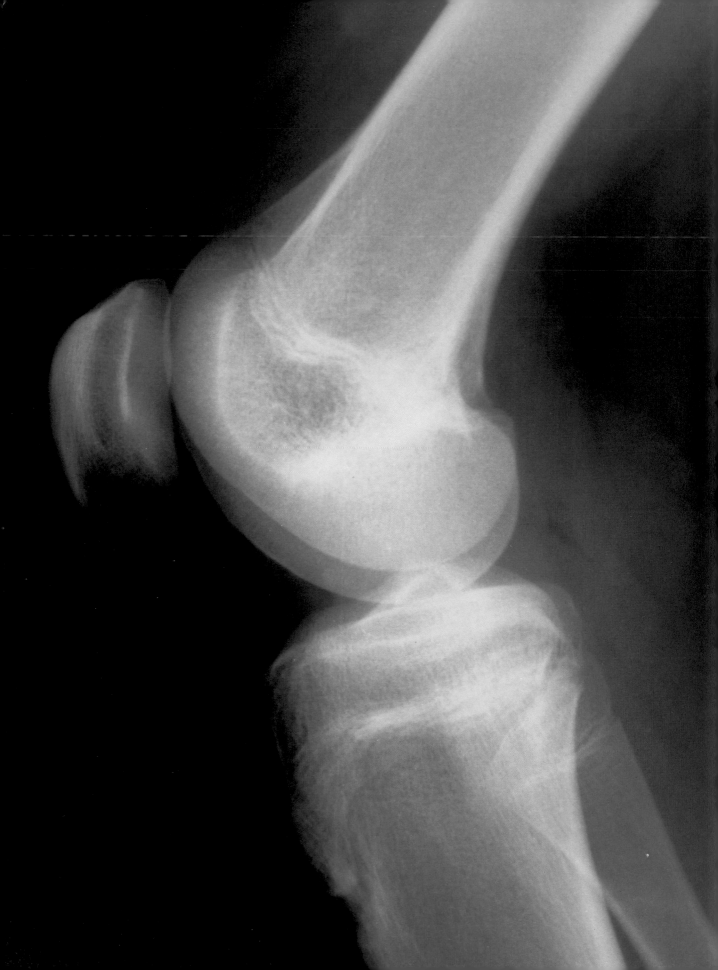

The Problem

Osteoporosis, the weakening and eventual breaking of bones, is often a silent, hidden problem until there is a sudden dramatic episode. Your arm, or your hip, may fracture or give way, and you become aware that something has gone wrong. Some people grow to fear osteoporosis as they get older, while others think it will never happen to them. Some people are totally oblivious to its existence, and this is quite understandable because there are often no overt symptoms to give you an early warning.

Understanding Osteoporosis

The word osteoporosis is derived from the Greek words *osteon* (bone) and *poros* (passageway, pore). It is often used as a catch-all for all disorders involving faulty or weakening bone structures, but there are actually three main problems – osteoporosis, osteomalacia and rickets – that may affect the bones within this concept.

Osteoporosis

Osteoporosis is defined as an absolute decrease in the total amount of bone-tissue mass, the remaining amount of bone being normal. The small structures that form the bone matrix gradually become smaller and thinner, and the spaces between them increase. As a result, bones become weaker, less dense and more porous. Small crush fractures occur from time to time, and gradually bone damage increases. The bones become progressively more fragile and more prone to breaking.

There are two types of specialized bone cells. Osteoblasts are bone-building cells; osteoclasts break down old bone material. These two cell types normally act in harmony with each other, and your bones remain healthy as old bone is broken down by the osteoclasts and new bone is built by the osteoblasts.

When osteoporosis occurs, this balance is altered in favour of the osteoclasts, and there is progressive bone breakdown. This is made worse if the intake of calcium from your diet is inadequate for the needs of the various cells in your body and if the level of calcium in your blood falls. When your diet contains an insufficient supply of calcium, the body compensates for the lowered levels in the blood by drawing the necessary calcium from the bones.

In other words, in osteoporosis, osteoblast (bone-building) activity continues as normal but osteoclasts (bone-breakdown) work overtime, removing calcium from bones and returning it to the blood. The whole process is accelerated when your intake of calcium is inadequate.

Types of osteoporosis

The two most common forms are Types 1 and 2; less common is secondary osteoporosis. The concept of types 1 and 2, though rarely used, does help to distinguish between symptom patterns.

- Type 1 is post-menopausal osteoporosis, which is thought to be brought about by the hormonal and other related changes that occur in women during the menopause.
- Type 2 is a gradual and progressive osteoporosis, which is age-related, affects both sexes and can start at any age.
- Secondary osteoporosis is caused by, and is secondary to, some other health problem, including hormonal problems, such as hypercortisonism and hypogonadism, partial gastrectomy (stomach removal) and multiple myeloma.

In both Type 1 and Type 2 osteoporosis (see box above) the balance between osteoblast and osteoclast activity is unbalanced, and the osteoclastic activity becomes dominant, thus weakening the bones.

Type 1

Type 1 osteoporosis is characterized by considerable bone loss in the spine. Typically, oestrogen levels will have fallen, and this lack of oestrogen leads to reduced output of a hormone called calcitonin (see page 24). The lack of calcitonin means that bone cells are allowed to break down too readily and leads to decreased production of the active form of vitamin D. Lack of vitamin D activity leads to reduced absorption of calcium from the digestive tract, and can lead to a loss of up to half your bone mass. At the same time, a lack of oestrogen leads to increased activity of the important parathyroid hormone (see page 23), which pulls calcium from your bones into the bloodstream.

Type 2

In type 2 osteoporosis in addition to the loss of bone in the spine, there is also loss in the bones of the rest of the body. Weaknesses are most likely to show up in the long bones of the legs and arms. This type of osteoporosis results from the gradual changes that occur with age, such as a decline in the quality and mineral content of the diet and a decline in the body's ability to synthesize vitamin D and to absorb calcium, magnesium and other necessary nutrients. These changes lead to increased activity of the parathyroid gland, and the increased amount of parathyroid hormone pulls calcium from the bones throughout the body. The bones become weakened, and widespread osteoporosis develops.

Osteomalacia

Osteomalacia, a word derived from *osteon* (bone) and *malakos* (soft), occurs in adults and involves a gradual loss of the elements calcium and phosphorus from the bones. The bones gradually become softer and more curved or bent, and there is an increased tendency for fractures to occur. Inadequate intake or availability of vitamin D is often a major contributing factor. The problem may also occur after several pregnancies when the body has been depleted of calcium and there has been insufficient vitamin D to assist the necessary replacement.

Although this book is about osteoporosis, in practical terms it applies to osteomalacia as well, because many of the solutions to the first problem will also help to improve the second.

Rickets

Rickets is similar to osteomalacia but occurs in children. Because their bones are in the process of growing, the changes are more immediately obvious than they would be in adults. Instead of a gradual breakdown of bones that were once well formed, bones that are affected by rickets are poorly formed from the start. This bone deformation leads to the well-known 'bow legs' as the growing bones

are not able to bear the full weight of the developing body. The forehead bulges and there is distortion of other bones of the head. In the chest there are signs of the condition known as a rachitic rosary, when the junctions of the ribs with the rib cartilage are distorted by a build-up of uncalcified tissue as the body attempts to compensate for the loss of available calcium.

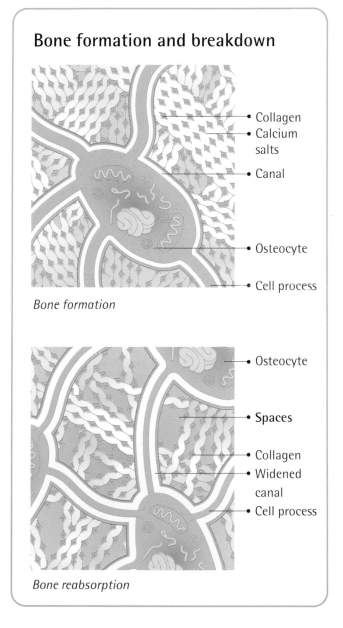

Bone formation and breakdown

• Collagen
• Calcium salts

• Canal

• Osteocyte

• Cell process

Bone formation

• Osteocyte

• Spaces

• Collagen
• Widened canal
• Cell process

Bone reabsorption

The extent of the problem

Osteoporosis is a major health risk, causing a huge drain on health services and often leading to serious disability or death. In Britain, for example:

- one in three women develop osteoporosis
- one in 12 men develop osteoporosis
- osteoporosis causes 200,000 bone fractures a year, of which 70,000 are hip fractures
- between 15 and 20 per cent of people die within six months of their osteoporosis-induced 'accident' making osteoporosis as big a killer as breast cancer
- fractures leave many people dependent on outside care to provide at least some of their needs, thereby fundamentally altering their lifestyle and also incurring great costs to health services
- the problem can cause debilitating and chronic pain, particularly in the back, can lead to a bent, stooped posture and a protruding abdomen, and can hasten ageing

How osteoporosis develops

Osteoporosis was a lot less common in earlier generations. Although the incidence of osteoporosis rises with age, and although the average age of the population is increasing, this is not the sole reason for the increase. More people are developing osteoporosis at a younger and younger age. This poses the following questions: Why has it increased in the past few decades? What differences are there in our lifestyles that have led to this increase?

We now know that osteoporotic changes, particularly of the spine, can start several years before the menopause in many women. Indeed, it is believed that half the total bone loss may have already occurred before a woman's level of oestrogen has fallen, which means that the menopause cannot be the only cause of osteoporosis. We used to lament the accident – the misplaced step or trip – that caused an elderly person, usually a woman, to fall and break a hip or a leg, but it is now thought more likely that a possible slight stress on bones that were already fragile caused a fracture. The fall, in effect, was a consequence of the break and not the cause.

In light of this, it is extremely important that your bones should remain strong throughout your life and particularly into old age. It is possible to have tests to monitor the strength of your bones. Prevention is always better than cure, and simple urine tests can pick up early warning signs long before any bone weakness will show on an x-ray. You should also find out how you can maintain the strength and structure of your bones. Finally, once you know what to do, make sure you actually do it. Too many people know what they should do and pay lip service to the need for action, but fail to make the necessary lifestyle changes.

Problem areas

Hip fractures are dramatic, life-changing events, but other areas of the body are also affected by osteoporosis, the second most frequent one being the spine or back. Many people complain of having an aching back without being aware that the pain may be caused by disintegrating

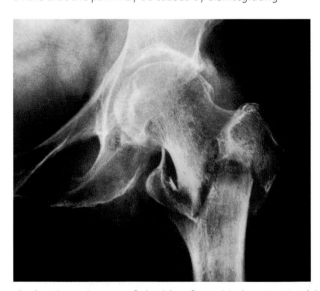

▲ A coloured x-ray of the hip of an elderly woman with a fractured femur caused by osteoporosis. This is signified by the red area around the joint.

Facts about osteoporosis

o Bone mass in the body reaches its peak during young adulthood.

o After a period of stability, from the age of about 40 there is a slow but steady loss of bone.

o Osteoporosis can occur at any time of your life, but usually from around 30 years of age onwards. It becomes overwhelmingly more common with increasing age and is associated with a progressive decrease in bone density.

o It does not, as is often assumed, necessarily start at or during the menopause.

Bone fracture risk factors

It is widely assumed that the greater the degree of osteoporosis the greater the risk of fracturing a bone. There are, however, many other factors that may be even more closely associated with a high risk of bone fracture. These include:

o the use of drugs, such as sleeping pills, tranquillizers and nicotine

o hormonal problems, such as an overactive thyroid gland

o a tall, slim physique

o poor visual depth perception

o a fast heartbeat

Women with all five of these risk factors have a 10 per cent chance of fracturing a bone in the next five years compared to a 1 per cent chance for a woman with two or fewer of these risk factors. This means that using osteoporosis as a guide to whether you are likely to break a bone is not necessarily reliable.

To assess your risk of fracturing a bone you would be better to use age and the strength of your muscles as a guide, and because there is little you can do about your age you should see what you can do to make sure that your muscle strength increases as you get older.

This means that you should undertake regular checks to make sure that you are not developing osteoporosis. You should avoid becoming complacent and should ensure that you regularly use your muscles to keep them strong.

vertebrae. The problem may not be as immediately obvious as a broken hip, but the pain and disability can be just as devastating and life-changing. A persistent back problem is not only painful but exhausting; it is inhibiting and often relentless, affecting both mood and behaviour. You might avoid going to social functions because you need to lie down at intervals to get relief. You might give up going to concerts or on outings because it is difficult to sit still for long periods. Back problems reduce your flexibility and often mean that lifting even light objects is a problem, and that bending down is either difficult or impossible.

The same is true of neck problems. The gradual osteoporotic weakening of the neck can lead to much pain and discomfort, and this is worsened if there has been a previous injury. An old whiplash injury, for instance, may well come back to haunt you when, years later, the vertebrae of your neck are further weakened by the development of osteoporosis. You may have thought soon after the event that the injury was not serious and that you had regained nearly all the movement of your neck. Several years later, however, you may find yourself wishing that you had taken better care of your bones at the time.

It is worth remembering that by the end of their lives men have generally lost 20–30 per cent of their bone mass and that the figure for women is 40–50 per cent. There is hope, however, and it is worth bearing in mind that osteoporosis is not inevitable, it can be avoided and even reversed, with:

• dietary and lifestyle management

• the use of nutritional and other supplements

• well-chosen exercises

The Skeleton

The Skeleton

The illustration below highlights the bones of the body that can be affected by osteoporosis. As a general rule it is usually the bigger bones, in the legs, that are most affected.

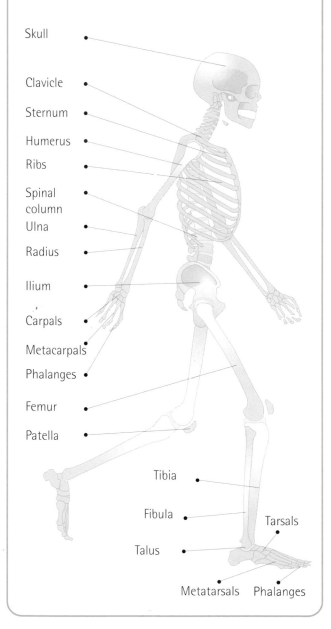

Skull

Clavicle

Sternum

Humerus

Ribs

Spinal column

Ulna

Radius

Ilium

Carpals

Metacarpals

Phalanges

Femur

Patella

Tibia

Fibula

Tarsals

Talus

Metatarsals   Phalanges

When people think of osteoporosis they tend to think of weak and crumbling bones, and when they think of bones they tend to think of solid tissue made mainly of calcium. The truth is rather different, and the structure of bone is actually quite complex. In addition to calcium, bones are made up of considerable amounts of organic matter and many minerals. They contain cells and fibrous connective material as well as the mineral bone mass, and require a number of vitamins and minerals for their formation, maintenance and general function.

The skeletal system

Your skeletal system makes up 10 per cent of your body. It includes all the bones in your body, which range in shape from the nearly spherical ones of your skull and the long, thin ones of your limbs to the flatter ones of your pelvis and the small, chunky ones that make up your wrist and ankle joints. Your skeleton also includes the joints that are formed as these bones attach to and move over and against each other..

This combination of bones and joints is made up of three types of tissue:
• the bones themselves: the entire bone mass, which consists of minerals, cells and the substances between them
• cartilage: the tough, flexible tissue that sits between and around bones and connects many of them together (think of the 'gristle' in a joint of meat and the fibres that hold the various bones together)
• hemopoietic tissue: the tissue, such as bone marrow, that occupies cavities within bones and produces blood cells

It is the bones themselves that are of concern to us here. It is important to keep in mind that your bones are in a constant state of dynamic equilibrium, and any lifestyle changes you make can have a positive or negative effect on them at any age.

What bones do

The skeleton performs five main functions:

Support

You need a skeleton so that you can stand up. Your bones define your overall structure, and it is from this structure or framework that all the other tissues and organs of your body are suspended.

Protection

Your bones protect many of your soft tissues. Your skull protects your brain, your rib cage protects your lungs and heart, and your pelvic girdle protects the internal organs that lie within it.

Movement

Your bones and their joints operate as a system of levers. They also provide anchorage for your muscles. As your muscles relax and contract, leverage is applied to the various bones and movement does or does not occur.

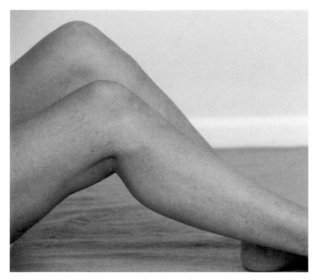

▲ Osteoporosis affects the bones of the skeleton. Damage to these bones will affect your general movement and mobility and can cause great upheaval to everyday life.

Bone formation and breakdown

The dynamic and parallel activities of building up new bone and breaking down old bone are necessary because:
- they enable your bones to grow and change shape
- they make it possible for old bone tissue to be replaced by new tissue
- they enable minerals to be released from bones when they are needed

In adult bones the cells (see page 16) make up between 1 and 5 per cent of the total bone mass.

Blood formation

Some bones contain either red or yellow bone marrow. Red bone marrow is responsible for making most of your blood cells; yellow bone marrow acts as a fat storage depot.

Mineral storage

The mineral part of your bones provides a place to store a certain amount of spare minerals. It provides, for instance, a calcium reservoir for the rest of your body. Other cells that need calcium can take it from your blood, and when, as a result, your blood calcium level falls, calcium can be drawn from your bones to bring the blood level back up to normal. When your blood calcium is high, such as can occur after a calcium-rich meal, the extra calcium can be re-deposited within your bones.

What bones are made of

When asked, most people say that their bones are made of calcium. In fact, this is far from the truth and, chemically, would be impossible. Calcium, a positive ion, needs a partner, a negative ion, to bond with, so, at most, your bones could be half calcium. The next most frequent answer is that 'bones are made of calcium carbonate, you know, like chalk'. But think about a piece of blackboard chalk and how easily it can be snapped. Your bones need to be much stronger than that.

In fact, the mineral part of your bones is a complex substance called hydroxyapatite (see opposite), but this makes up only a part of the whole structure. Like all the other tissues in your body, your bones are made up of three main components:
- cells: which produce most of the other material of the tissue
- interconnecting fibrous material: which holds the tissue together
- intercellular matrix: which fills the gaps between these two

Cells

The specialized cells within your bones are called osteocytes, from *osteon* (bone) and *kutos* (vessel, receptacle). As we have seen (on page 10), there are two types of osteocytes: osteoblasts, cells that help to build up new bones, and osteoclasts, cells that are responsible for the breakdown of old and worn-out bone cells.

Interconnecting material

The connective tissue is produced by cells in the tissue. In bones this connective tissue consists mainly of collagen, which is made up of long, thin protein chains that are arranged in bundles and form fibres. They are embedded in a firm gel and, rather like the metal rods in reinforced concrete (the intercellular matrix, see below), add to the strength of your bones.

Intercellular matrix

The third component of bones is the intercellular matrix. This is the ground substance that fills up all the spaces between the cells and the collagen so that the cells are embedded in it and the connective tissue fibres pass through it. This material is also made by the bone cells and consists, initially, of complex organic material.
Bones, therefore, at this stage, consist entirely of organic matter, not calcium, and it is only after the matrix of the bone has been formed that it is calcified or hardened as the various minerals – mainly, but not exclusively, calcium – are laid down within it. The bones of babies contain relatively more collagen and less calcium than those of an adult. As infants grow, the amount of calcium deposited in their bones increases, and the bones become progressively harder and stronger and more able to take the toddlers' weight as they start to crawl or walk. It is important to keep in mind that the strength of your bones could not be achieved without the presence of the connective tissues that interpenetrate the matrix, resembling, as we have seen, the reinforcing rods in the concrete (mineral) matrix.

Finally, bones also contain blood vessels, which pass through the tissue, taking oxygen and nutrients to the bones and aiding the removal of toxins and waste products. From all this it should be clear that the structure of bones

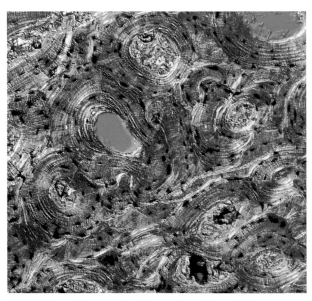

▲ *A light micrograph of a section through human compact bone. Compact bone is structured into concentric bone layers (lamellae) arranged around channels, seen here as clear areas, containing blood, lymph vessels and nerves.*

is complex and is made up of a range of components, both inorganic and organic. It is not surprising, therefore, that many different substances are needed for the formation of bones. Not only do we need minerals, we also need proteins, vitamins, which play a part in the catalyst systems that aid in both the formation and functioning of bones, and hormones, which control and affect the way bones function.

Mineral components

As noted earlier, the main mineral component of bones is hydroxyapatite. There are also certain amounts of calcium carbonate and smaller amounts of other minerals.

Hydroxyapatite is a combination of calcium and phosphorus within which are spaces for other minerals or metal ions. Some of the calcium within this structure is replaced by magnesium, which adds to the strength of bones. Sometimes calcium is replaced by sodium, potassium and other elements. Phosphorus may be replaced by other non-metal ions, such as citrate, bicarbonate, fluoride and chloride.

There is a further, less healthy, possibility. If you are exposed to toxic metals, such as lead, these may enter and be retained by the bones, as they are able to be taken into spaces left by calcium. If you are calcium-deficient, therefore, and there are empty calcium spaces in the hydroxyapatite mineral lattice of your bones, and if, at the same time, you are exposed to toxic lead ions, you will take up and absorb more lead than you would if you were not calcium-deficient.

The two major components of hydroxyapatite, calcium and phosphorus, form an approximately alternating matrix and are present in ratios that vary between 1.4:1 and 2.1:1. This mineralization of the matrix is responsible for the hardness of bone. The overall construction of bones in general and the organization of hydroxyapatite in particular have evolved to give the maximum amount of strength to bones for their weight-bearing function for the minimum amount of weight and mass.

The total bone structure as described previously makes up healthy bones, strong enough to carry the weight of your body, yet flexible enough to withstand the bumps and bangs of daily life. Without its inorganic, calcium-rich hydroxyapatite, bone would maintain its overall shape and structure but would be as flexible as tendon and would be unable to support your body's weight. On the other hand, bone that consisted only of calcium- and phosphorus-rich hydroxyapatite, but no organic matter, would also maintain its shape, but it would be fragile and brittle, breaking easily when tapped or hit.

Bone-coating tissue

Your bones are surrounded by layers of sensitive tissue called endosteum and periosteum, which form thin skins around your bones. If you look carefully at the bones in a piece of meat you will be able to see them. They are important and sensitive tissues, containing a number of nerve cells. When you bump or break a bone it is not, in the main, the bone itself that hurts, for bone does not contain the type of sensory nerve cells that register pain. Most of the pain comes from the nerve cells in the periosteum that coats the bones.

When a child suffers from 'growing pains' it is generally because a bone is growing faster than its surrounding endosteum and periosteum, and it is the stretching of these tissues that causes the pain. Parents are usually told that the child will 'grow out of it'. In other words, with time the periosteum will grow in proportion to the bone and the pain will stop. The problem can generally be solved simply, and much more rapidly, by supplying increased amounts of the nutrients needed by these tissues for their normal growth, and two of the necessary nutrients commonly lacking in this regard are zinc and manganese.

Symptoms and Diagnosis

Who is most at risk?

Osteoporosis is more common:
- among women than men
- among post-menopausal than pre-menopausal women
- in women who weigh less than 50kg (110lb, 7st 12oz) than in heavier women
- in developed countries than in developing ones
- among city-dwellers than country-dwellers
- among white women than black women
- in countries where the diet contains a significant proportion of milk, cheese and other dairy products than in countries where the consumption of dairy products is small or non-existent

This last point is of particular interest, and we will be considering it in greater detail later (see page 59). It is also interesting to note that there are some countries in which osteoporosis is very rare.

Most white women over the age of 70 have a one in four chance of being hospitalized for broken bones, and when osteoporosis occurs in men it is most likely to be found in older men who are also heavy drinkers. Finally, right-handed people are more likely to break the less used bones on the left side of their bodies.

Symptoms

Osteoporosis, generally, is a silent killer. For many years, while your bones are diminishing in density and strength, you may experience no symptoms at all. This is unfortunate, because it means there are no early warning signs until the osteoporotic process is far advanced. Often, the first indication of the problem is when you suffer a fracture, yet the consequences can be severe, life-changing and even life-threatening. Remember

that Type 1 osteoporosis, which is common among post-menopausal women, is most likely to involve the back. Over time, pain – which can often be low-level, mild back pain – may develop. Other symptoms may then appear.

1 There may be a growing number of incidences of acute pain. You may do something that puts slightly more pressure than usual on your back, such as picking up a heavy object. It may be something you used to be able to pick up easily and safely, but suddenly you find that this effort causes you an acute and stabbing or sharp pain as a crush fracture occurs. If you are lucky this will be felt as a dull ache for a few days and then clear up as the bone struggles to repair itself. If it happens several times or is severe, the pain is likely to get worse and to continue for longer; it is also likely to recur when you put a similar strain, even a very mild one, on the same place. Eventually, a persistent back problem may develop.

2 If several vertebrae are involved, the spine will become misshapen and you could develop a 'dowager's hump', the instantly recognizable hump at the top of the back. The top of the spine becomes curved, and the typical bent-over posture leaves the sufferer staring at the ground, unable to look up or even, in extreme cases, to look straight ahead. It is often associated with pain and with loss of height. Even without this curvature and hump, you may lose a few centimetres in height.

Prime Candidate

If we were to develop the prototype of the sort of person who is most at risk of developing osteoporosis, we would have a post-menopausal white woman, who lives in a city in a Western country and who eats dairy products and what we might call the 'typical' Western diet.

3 For some people the first indication that they have osteoporosis may come as the result of an x-ray, possibly taken for some other purpose.

4 In Type 2 osteoporosis develops gradually with increasing age. The areas most likely to be affected include the hips, forearms and wrists as well as the back. In practice, there is commonly an overlap of both types in susceptible people – that is, women as they age and reach the menopause – and so the results can be detected in both the back and the limbs.

Diagnosis

Many different methods of detection are available, although not all are ideal, and some are problematic. They indicate osteoporosis only once it has developed to a considerable extent.

Blood tests can be used to check a number of factors, including calcium and phosphate levels, the level of alkaline phosphatase (an enzyme involved in bone metabolism) and the amount of vitamin D3 or 1:25DHCC (calciferol, the active form of vitamin D). Unfortunately, none of these measurements is specific for osteoporosis. Low blood calcium could mean simply that there has been an inadequate intake, but it may not mean that there is (yet) any osteoporosis. Altered levels of alkaline phosphatese could indicate increased bone activity or turnover, but this could also be an indication of other problems, such as Paget's disease or bone cancer. A raised erythrocyte sedimentation rate (ESR) is used to detect arthritis or rheumatism, but it indicates inflammation and is not useful in the prediction of osteoporosis.

Blood tests are really useful only for detecting secondary osteoporosis, not primary osteoporosis. However, the information derived from blood tests, when combined with information from other diagnostic tools, can improve the overall assessment.

X-rays can be helpful but only in detecting osteoporosis when it is relatively far advanced. They can show decreased vertebral bone density, but the structures become changed as the problem progresses, and their subjective assessment is open to error.

Other types of scans are available, including dual energy x-ray absorptiometry (DEXA). This is non-invasive and rapid. It uses a low level of radiation and assesses bone density at specific at-risk locations, such as the lumbar spine, the top of the femur (thigh bone) and the lower arm. It can be used to document your current skeletal density and risk of fracture, and is useful in monitoring the efficacy of therapy.

The ideal test would be one that picked up the problem when it was beginning to develop. If you could detect the start of osteoporotic change, you could do something about it before it developed further. There are now two tests that may help to achieve this. Both involve measuring the amounts of collagen markers present in urine. These substances are lost from bones into the bloodstream and from there into urine during bone reabsorption or bone breakdown. The more of these compounds that show up in your urine the more likely you are to be developing osteoporosis. In other words, these tests show when a person has started to develop an osteoporotic pattern of bone metabolism. They distinguish between people who are rapid losers and those who are slow losers of bone mass, and they also show this in appreciable time before there are visual osteoporotic changes in bone structure. Obviously, if you are a fast loser you are more at risk of developing osteoporosis than if you are a slow loser.

If these tests show that bone reabsorption is starting to occur, it is time to start a serious prevention programme. Do not wait for the osteoporosis to develop fully.

Risk Factors

There are many possible causes of osteoporosis. Unfortunately, attention has focused on only two of them: an inadequate intake of calcium and low levels of the hormone oestrogen. There are, however, many others, and these must also be taken into account. As we consider them, start to think about the ones that could apply to you and what you can do about them.

It is important to do all you can to determine the cause of your osteoporosis, existing or potential, for two reasons. First, when you know what is causing the problem you can make appropriate changes so that it does not continue. Second, knowing the cause will often point to steps you can take to treat the problem and possibly reverse the situation. Focusing solely on a possible lack of adequate calcium intake and the need for more oestrogen, as many women do, may mean that you are overlooking useful information that could be helping you to improve the state of your bones.

Calcium

The loss of calcium from bones can occur because of one or more of the following:

• a lack of calcium in the diet
• a reduced absorption of calcium from the digestive system
• a reduced deposition of calcium in bones
• an increased loss of calcium from bones

These problems generally worsen with age. Although the diet of most people, no matter what their age, is generally deficient in calcium, the nutritional quality of people's diet often deteriorates with age and thus contains progressively less calcium. This is particularly true of people who live alone if they decide that it is too much trouble to cook a proper meal 'for just one person' and so resort to snacks and sandwiches. In addition, with age, the body's digestive system functions less efficiently, and people may find it increasingly difficult to absorb minerals, including calcium.

Causes of low levels of calcium

• Lack of calcium in the diet.
• Lack of appropriate supplements.
• Lack of proper calcium absorption.
• Low level of stomach acid.
• Insufficient vitamin D.
• Lack of digestive enzymes.
• Poor liver function and bile flow.
• Poor pancreatic function.
• Intestinal problems, such as candidiasis, parasites, putrefaction and damaged intestinal walls (leading to poor absorption).
• Constipation.

The problem is much more complex than this, however, because even the absorption of calcium is not a straightforward process. It is relatively simple for the body to absorb vitamins because, with the exception of vitamin B12, they are small organic molecules which can cross the walls of the intestinal tract relatively easily. Minerals, on the other hand, are inorganic molecules, which are not at home in the organic matrix of body tissues, and for this reason their absorption is less easy and depends on a number of factors within the digestive tract.

Calcium absorption requires an adequate production of acid by the cells of the stomach. Unfortunately, many people, even those who experience heartburn and related digestive problems, actually produce an insufficient amount of this acid, and the amount that is produced generally decreases with age.

The body must also produce the appropriate digestive enzymes from the pancreas and bile from the liver. Otherwise, undigested fats can bind with calcium and the complex is lost from the body in the faeces.

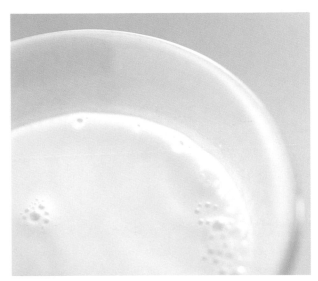

▲ *When calcium is mentioned everybody immediately thinks of milk and, as you will discover in subsequent chapters, this is not necessarily the best source.*

Carrier molecules within the walls of the small intestine pick up the minerals from the intestine and carry them across to the other side. Calcium and other minerals are released by these intestinal carrier molecules and enter the bloodstream where, as often as not, other carrier molecules transport them throughout the body. The correct absorption and utilization of calcium within the body also depends on the presence of vitamin D (see

Causes of low levels of phosphorus

○ A deficiency of phosphates in the diet (this is not common).
○ A far greater proportion of phosphorus to calcium in the diet (a ratio greater than 1:1).
○ A far greater proportion of calcium to phosphorus in the diet (this is not common).
○ Inadequate availability of vitamin D.
○ The typical Western diet.

page 23). Reduced levels of calcium can, therefore, have a number of causes (see box, left).

Phosphorus

Phosphorus is the second most common mineral element in the body, and 80 per cent of it occurs in bones and teeth as part of the mineral hydroxyapatite. In bones calcium is partnered by phosphate, a combination of phosphorus and oxygen, and it is important that both phosphorus and calcium are consumed in approximately equal proportions. The absorption of phosphorus, like that of calcium, depends on the presence in the body of the active form of vitamin D.

An excessive intake of phosphorus, a relatively common occurrence, is a recognized factor in the development of osteoporosis because it can increase the excretion of calcium from the body. Conversely, an excess intake of calcium compared to phosphorus (a relatively rare occurrence) can lead to the increased excretion of phosphate. It is generally suggested that the intake of the two should be approximately equal, although it is interesting to note that the ratio of calcium to phosphorus in cows' milk is 1.2:1, whereas the ratio in human milk is 2:1, so that human milk provides twice as much calcium as phosphorus.

Unfortunately, the typical diet of most people in the Western world consists largely of foods that are high in phosphorus and low in calcium. This, by its very nature, is more likely to lead to osteoporosis than a more traditional diet, typically found in rural communities and developing countries. It is no surprise, therefore, to find that osteoporosis is most common in Western countries.

A diet that contains a disproportionately large amount of phosphorus compared with calcium can cause the parathyroid gland to become overactive and lead to increased leaching of calcium from bones. This occurs no matter how much calcium you consume.

Magnesium

More than two-thirds of the magnesium in your body is present in the bones, where it is an essential part of the structure. Magnesium can mimic calcium and enter calcium spaces in the hydroxyapatite crystal (see page 17), and it is desirable that it does do so.

Magnesium is absorbed from the small intestine in the same way that calcium is. In fact, the two elements compete with each other for absorption, and it is, therefore, important that they are consumed in the correct proportions – you need up to twice as much calcium as magnesium. What this means for your diet is discussed on page 56.

It is important to note that, if you have been prescribed or are taking a calcium supplement for your health and the prevention or treatment of osteoporosis, it is also important that you take an approximately equivalent amount of magnesium. Unfortunately, this recommendation is often overlooked.

Causes of low levels of magnesium

o Inadequate intake of magnesium.
o Incorrect ratio of calcium to magnesium in the diet or in supplements.
o Inadequate vitamin D.

Aluminium

Aluminium is a toxic metal, which enters the body from a number of sources. First, traces can be ingested from equipment, such as aluminium saucepans, utensils, cans or foil. Second, it can be present in food. It is, for example, added to salt to make it flow freely, to baking powder and to maraschino cherries. Third, it is a constituent of many antacid medications and is applied to the skin in many antiperspirants and deodorants.

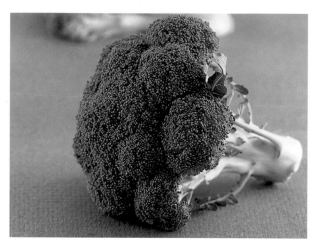

▲ *Food such as broccoli, Brussels sprouts, spinach and cabbage contain high levels of magnesium (see charts on page 122–25 for more information).*

Aluminium can have an adverse effect on your bones by means of its action on phosphorus and calcium. If it is present in the intestinal tract it can bind with inorganic phosphorus, which means that the phosphorus is not available for absorption and is lost from the body in the faeces. Since, as we have seen, most people consume too much phosphorus and not enough calcium and since the relative amounts of the two are important, this might not seem to be a bad thing. However, phosphorus also takes calcium and fluoride with it from the intestinal tract.

Aluminium in the body is associated with senility, loss of memory and an inability to concentrate, so it is important that its intake is minimized. Do not use aluminium saucepans or other aluminium cookware; do not use aluminium foil; do not drink liquids from lightweight

Causes of ingestion of aluminium

o Consumption of aluminium in food and drink.
o Absorption via the skin.
o Ingestion in medication.

aluminium cans; and do not eat food that contains added aluminium. Although you may do all you can to avoid the use of aluminium utensils at home, when you eat in restaurants you are almost certain to be eating food that has been cooked in or prepared with aluminium equipment.

Vitamin D

Vitamin D is, as we have seen, critical for the correct absorption and utilization of calcium and phosphorus. You obtain vitamin D in two ways: from your diet or by making it under your skin. In the diet it comes largely from the livers of fish (cod liver oil or halibut liver oil), or of calves or chicken, from eggs and the fatty part of dairy products, such as cream, butter and cheese. In the skin it is made by the action of sunlight falling on a derivative of cholesterol.

Whether it is consumed or made, vitamin D has to be altered into its active form. It goes first to the liver, where it is converted into 25HCC; this goes to the kidneys and is converted into its active form, 1:25DHCC, which works with parathyroid hormone, one of the two hormones that have a powerful effect on calcium metabolism and bones.

It is worth knowing how vitamin D acts in the body so that we understand that simply taking a vitamin D supplement may not be enough. If your liver or kidneys are not working properly the conversion of any vitamin D you consume to its fully active form will be impeded.

Causes of low levels of vitamin D

- Inadequate intake of vitamin D.
- Inadequate sun exposure for the production of vitamin D.
- Poor liver function.
- Poor kidney function.

Some people have to have injections of the active form, 1:25DHCC, because their bodies cannot produce enough. Looking after your liver and kidneys is, therefore, a sensible part of preventing osteoporosis. However, even this may not be enough, and you may need help from your doctor.

Hormones

Parathyroid hormone

Parathyroid hormone (PTH) and calcitonin (see page 24) are two key hormones in the metabolism of calcium. They work together, but in opposite ways. PTH is secreted from your parathyroid glands in response to low levels of calcium in your blood. When the calcium level in your blood falls, the hormone acts in three ways to bring it back to normal. These three actions raise the level of calcium in the blood to normal:

- it increases the amount of calcium that is absorbed across the intestinal walls from dietary intake by increasing the conversion of 25HCC to 1:25DHCC in the kidneys (see vitamin D, opposite)
- it acts directly on the kidneys to inhibit or block the loss of calcium from the body in urine
- if the first two methods are insufficient, it draws calcium from the bones

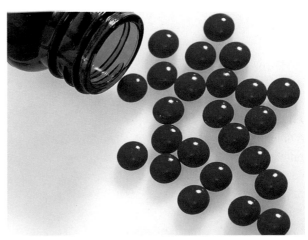

▲ *If you cannot get sufficient levels of vitamin D from your diet it may be worth considering supplementation.*

A lack of PTH will reduce your ability to absorb calcium and could contribute to osteoporosis. Be aware that in vitamin D deficiency, as in rickets or osteomalacia, there is little PTH can do to increase calcium absorption; blood calcium levels are maintained because calcium is drawn from bones.

Risk facts associated with parathyroid hormone

o A low parathyroid function will affect the metabolism of calcium.
o The condition may be worsened by a lack of vitamin D and/or a lack of calcium.

Calcitonin

The hormone calcitonin is produced by your thyroid gland in response to a rise in blood calcium level, therefore working in opposition to PTH. It does this by increasing the activity of the osteoblasts thus depositing calcium in bones. It also inhibits the action of osteoclasts and so holds calcium in bones.

If your calcium intake is inadequate or if your blood calcium level never rises above normal, as it would after a high intake of calcium, calcitonin will not be stimulated into activity. A lack of calcitonin is worrying as it could mean that you fail to deposit calcium in your bones, even when it is present in the bloodstream in an adequate amount.

Possible effects of insufficient calcitonin

o A failure of calcitonin metabolism.
o A lack of calcium.

Oestrogen

Oestrogen, one of the female hormones, is closely associated with calcium metabolism.

• It increases the formation of calcitonin.
• It stimulates the synthesis of the active forms of vitamin D and the absorption of calcium from the intestine.
• It is generally understood to slow down bone loss but to have only a limited effect on osteoblasts and so does little to stimulate new bone growth.

Oestrogen is not the most useful chemical in the body for stimulating bone growth; progesterone, ipriflavone and vitamin K are all more important. However, the publicity is focused on oestrogen. This has led to an assumption that the menopause, when a woman's oestrogen output falls, should be treated as a crisis, that doctors should be consulted and that replacement hormones should be taken. However, a consideration of a woman's life cycle suggests that this is not necessarily the case.

Before she reaches puberty, a girl cannot conceive, cannot bear a baby and does not need enhanced calcium absorption. She needs only to absorb sufficient calcium for herself and for her growing bones. At this time she produces a moderate amount of oestrogen.

At puberty, conception becomes possible and thus the possibility of the woman having to create a baby's skeleton arises. It is a useful metabolic development that the hormonal changes that lead to the body's being able to conceive and proceed with a pregnancy also encourage an increase in calcium absorption and availability.

After the menopause conception is no longer possible; the female body will not have to make another set of bones; so enhanced calcium absorption is no longer necessary. Thus it would seem that there is no need to worry. When the menopause occurs the resulting drop in oestrogen output and the lowered calcium absorption

Possible effects of insufficient oestrogen

- Inadequate intake and absorption of calcium
- Stress
- Adrenal fatigue

should leave the woman able to absorb all the calcium she needs for herself, now that child-bearing is no longer a possibility.

If this does not hold true, we have to ask ourselves how women managed for millions of years, when no oestrogen supplements were available. However, the theory is based on the assumption that throughout her life the woman has eaten an adequate diet, rich in calcium, magnesium and other minerals, and that she continues to do so after the menopause. Unfortunately, today's diet contains insufficient calcium, and the enhanced oestrogen levels

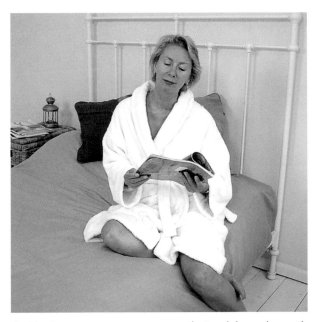

▲ *Most women are now aware that calcium absorption is linked to the level of oestrogen in the body.*

of a woman's fertile years are often needed simply to maintain the woman's own calcium level. Had she borne a child every year or two, as is biologically possible, it is likely that she would have become severely calcium-deficient. The diet of our ancient ancestors provided much more calcium than does today's average Western diet. It is in these circumstances that the reduced level of oestrogen production after the menopause increases the risk of osteoporosis. The problem is not so much the reduced oestrogen level but a prolonged inadequate intake of calcium. It would be better to have an adequate calcium intake throughout life than to take oestrogen supplements later.

- Oestrogen therapy must be taken for several years, usually ten or more, to get the full benefits.
- Considerable dangers result from taking oestrogen, including an increased risk of developing a number of types of cancer, including uterine and breast cancers.

The production of ovarian oestrogen is reduced at the menopause, but oestrogen continues to be produced from the adrenal glands provided they are not over-stressed.

Progesterone

Progesterone, another important female hormone, affects calcium metabolism and bone density. The levels change both at puberty and at or before the menopause, possibly as long as ten years before. Type 2 osteoporosis is progressive with age, can start many years before the menopause and may not be directly related to a fall in the production of oestrogen. Progesterone may be even more important than oestrogen in the prevention of osteoporosis. Thus the osteoporosis may be due to a deficiency of progesterone rather than a direct result of the menopause. Unlike oestrogen, progesterone may actually reverse some of the bone changes and contribute to an increase in bone density. Other studies, however, are not so convincing. There is much debate about which of the female sex hormones is the more important in relation to

Risk factors associated with progesterone

- Levels of oestrogen and progesterone can be altered.
- The menopause, particularly if the diet has been and is calcium-deficient.

osteoporosis and if taking either of them is worth any possible attendant risk. Nevertheless, many women have started to use a progesterone cream as a way of applying this hormone, and they believe it will produce better results than oestrogen. In a world where people want instant fixes and are unwilling to make significant changes to the way they live, it is tempting to use tablets, creams or injections. Yet there are risks. The lifestyle changes suggested in this book can make at least as great a difference to the health of your bones, possibly greater, and without any risk of adverse side effects.

Remember that all hormones are powerful compounds. They have profound effects on your body, acting on and instructing a variety of target organs and tissues to change the ways they behave. In addition to producing the results you desire, they may well, and often do, produce undesirable and even dangerous effects.

DHEA
DHEA (Dehydroepiandrosterone), a steroid hormone produced by the adrenal glands (see page 28), is relevant

Possible effects of insufficient DHEA

- Under-production of DHEA.
- Exhausted or tired adrenal glands.

to the state of the bones of both men and women, including post-menopausal women. The body's output of DHEA diminishes with age, and some studies have shown that the lower your serum or blood level of a DHEA derivative called DHEA-S, the greater is the likelihood that you are developing osteoporosis.

DHEA may help to prevent osteoporosis by:
- acting in a manner similar to oestrogen and inhibiting bone reabsorption
- stimulating bone formation and calcium absorption
- converting into oestrogen and testosterone

General health
The strength and mass of the bones you have in your early years largely depend on two factors, your genes and your environment.

Heredity, gender and environment
An obvious cause of osteoporosis is having poor bones from birth and through childhood and, if your genetic makeup is such that you have relatively large, dense bones you will be better off than someone with delicate, light bones. Because bone mass decreases slowly over the years, if your bones were weak or thin in your first decades, they are likely to reach fragile breaking point sooner than those of someone who started life with large, dense bones. This gives men an advantage over women. Men have heavier bones than women and they don't produce babies, so their bones will still be relatively dense even after the inevitable loss of bone mass that occurs with ageing.

You are fortunate if your diet was good throughout your childhood and if you enjoyed playing sports rather than spending all your time hunched over the latest book or computer game. However, you cannot hold your genes and your parents responsible for everything: you will have put yourself at greater risk if you chose to adopt a number of counterproductive habits, such as refusing to eat your vegetables and eating junk food instead. Smoking,

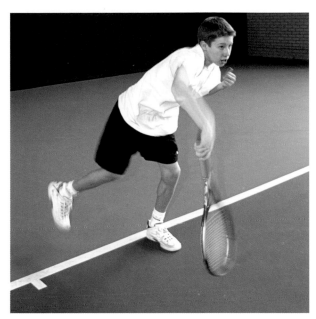

▲ *Enjoying sports as a child can actually be of great benefit to your bones later in life.*

drinking to excess and other such bad habits are also detrimental (see page 32–35).

Another aspect of heredity relates to how your ageing has been programmed genetically. The genetic makeup of some people is such that they lose bone mass faster than others. An unlucky few may even have a greatly accelerated rate of bone loss compared to others. This may have a number of causes, including an increased sensitivity to parathyroid hormone (see page 23).

Risk factors associated with heredity and environment

o Genetic factors include small bone size and rapid bone ageing.
o Environmental factors of childhood include low-calcium diet and minimal amounts of physical activity.

You may be tempted to think: 'If the problem is all in my genes there is nothing I can do about it and I might as well not bother trying.' This is not true. You cannot change your genetic makeup, of course, but you can work on the outcome and get the very best you can from of your genetic potential. The alternative is not to bother and to let any genetic disadvantages have full play, leading to the worst possible outcome.

The same is true of your childhood. You may feel like saying: 'Well, that's it then, my childhood got me off to a poor start, the damage is done and there's no hope for me now.' Again, this would be a mistake. No matter what your background, there are things you can do now to improve the outcome. If your background predisposed you to the problem, it is even more important to do all you can to stop or reverse the process.

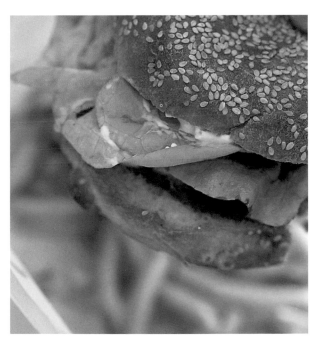

▲ *Eating junk food can have a very negative effect on your health; if you absolutely have to eat juicy hamburgers, make them healthy by using lean minced meat, adding crisp lettuce and tomatoes and combining it with a side-salad.*

Pregnancy

Being pregnant means creating a new human body with its associated demand for calcium and other nutrients. If you have borne one or more children you should consider the effects on your bone strength.

However, women possess additional adaptive mechanisms to enable them to absorb more than usual amounts of calcium from their diets during pregnancy and thus to be better able to provide the amounts needed for the foetus. In addition, many women consciously increase their calcium intake during pregnancy, either by improving their diet or by taking supplements. Some studies have suggested that multiple pregnancies may actually lower a woman's risk of developing fractures in later life.

Pregnancy and breast-feeding

Rather than thinking of pregnancy and breast-feeding as risk factors, it is important to understand the changes that occur at these times and to act appropriately.

Adrenal glands

The majority of a woman's oestrogen is produced in her ovaries, but additional oestrogen is produced elsewhere in the body, such as in some fatty tissues and, most importantly, in the adrenal glands. Men also produce some oestrogen in their adrenal glands throughout their lives. We have already noted the activity of the adrenal glands in many aspects of preventing osteoporosis, and it is important to understand how the glands function.

From the cortex (outer skin) your adrenal glands produce steroid hormones, such as oestrogen, progesterone, DHEA (see page 24-6), cortisone and others. These hormones have many functions – they balance sexual activity, control the metabolism of fats, proteins and

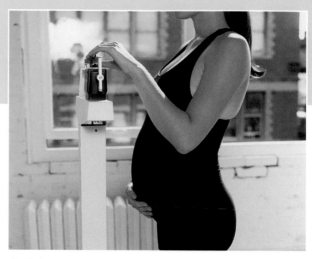

▲ *Being pregnant can place a huge demand on your body as it is having to provide enough calcium and nutrients for the baby and yourself, and you should consider the effects it can have on your bone strength.*

carbohydrates, boost your immune system and control fluid balance. They also help you to handle stress.

The medulla (the central part of the glands) produces the hormones adrenalin and noradrenalin, which, help you to handle stress. When a shock or alarm occurs adrenalin is pumped out into your body, where it acts to make your heart pump more strongly, your respiration rate to increase and your blood sugar level to rise so that a source of immediate energy is available to deal with the emergency. This is all well and good – it is perfectly normal – but if you are repeatedly under stress, if the stress is ongoing and you do not give your glands time to recover, problems can occur.

If you do not provide all the nutrients and care your glands need to keep on functioning, they can become exhausted, and when this happens their production of hormones is compromised. In the context of osteoporosis, this means that your alternative (if you are a woman) or your major (if you are a man) output of oestrogen is compromised. This, in turn, can increase your risk of developing osteoporosis. Give them generous amounts of all the B group vitamins, especially pantothenic acid (or calcium pantothenate if you are getting it from supplements). Reduce the stress in your life by any means you can and ensure that you have adequate periods of rest and relaxation.

Thyroid gland

Your thyroid gland is in the front of your neck and is responsible for controlling the rate at which food is metabolized and converted into energy or body fat. It also stimulates the activity of the osteoclasts that break down your bones. This reabsorption increases the level of calcium in your blood and decreases parathyroid activity and the availability of vitamin D in the body.

Thus, a high output of thyroid hormones, a condition known as hyperthyroidism, leads to reduced calcium absorption and increased bone breakdown and has been associated with an increased risk of developing osteoporosis. You will convert an excessive amount of food into energy, generate an excessive amount of heat and store a reduced amount of what you eat. This may sound like the answer to your prayers if you have spent years dieting, particularly if you are also lacking in energy. However, the apparent advantages are outweighed by a number of unwanted symptoms. People with an overactive thyroid gland often complain of finding it difficult to relax; they sweat a lot and are full of restless energy.

People with an underactive thyroid gland convert only a small amount of what they eat into energy, and the rest of their food all too easily adds those unwanted kilos or pounds to their stores of body fat. Other symptoms include weakness, dry or coarse skin, lethargy, slow speech, oedema (or swelling) of the eyelids, feeling cold, cold skin, reduced sweating, a thick tongue, facial oedema, coarseness of hair, an enlarged heart, pale skin, a poor

Risk factors associated with the thyroid gland

- A history of having had an overactive thyroid gland.
- An overactive thyroid gland at present.
- An excess of thyroid medication.

Thyroid function

- If your resting temperature is between 36.55–36.78°C (97.8–98.2°F) your thyroid gland is probably functioning normally.
- If your resting temperature is below 36.55°C (97.8°F) you probably have an underactive thyroid. The degree of underactivity may not be sufficient to produce serious clinical symptoms and negative signs on a blood test, but it could well be sufficient to cause fatigue and lack of energy.
- If your resting temperature is above 36.78°C (98.2°F) your thyroid gland is probably overactive and may be contributing to bone loss.

memory, constipation, weight gain, hair loss, pale lips, laboured or difficult breathing, swelling of the feet and hoarseness. There may also be additional symptoms, such as slow movements, muscle weakness, depression and burning or tingling sensations.

Having an overactive thyroid can be likened to having the central heating turned up too high so that everyone feels uncomfortably hot and sweaty. Having an underactive thyroid can be likened to having central heating thermostat set so low that everyone is shivering.

The normal medical treatment for hyperthyroidism is the surgical removal of part of the thyroid gland. The exact amount is hard to determine so a slightly larger section of the gland is removed and the shortfall in hormone output is made up by thyroid medication.

Post-menopausal women who have undergone partial thyroidectomy have reduced bone density whether or not they receive thyroxin medication afterwards, due either to the preceding period of overactivity or to excessive medication afterwards. If, as part of your treatment, you receive even a slight excess of thyroxin therapy it can lead to reduced bone mass and to osteoporosis. If you have ever had an overactive thyroid gland it would be wise to have tests done to determine the state of your bones.

If you think your thyroid gland is overactive speak to a professional and get advice. Keep in mind that an overactive thyroid gland, while possibly keeping you slightly slimmer and more energetic than you might otherwise be, is also overstressing your normal metabolism and is likely to increase your risk of getting osteoporosis. Your doctor may be able to help you if your thyroid gland is not functioning optimally, and a number of homoeopathic and naturopathic remedies are also available for this problem.

Testing your own thyroid function

You may be wondering about your own thyroid gland and whether it is functioning correctly.

There is a simple test that you can do at home that costs nothing and that will give you a more accurate answer than a blood test. All you need is a thermometer and some patience. The test involves measuring your temperature when you are as relaxed as you can possibly be. The best time to do this is usually when you have just woken up and are still dozing in bed. Prepare the thermometer the night before so it is ready to use.

Complete a normal temperature check when you are as relaxed as you can possibly be by placing a thermometer under your armpit. Repeat this process for about a week or ten days and keep a record of the results. If you are a man or women you can take this test in any group of convenient days. However, please bear in mind that if you are female and are between puberty and the menopause you should, ideally, start on the second or third day of menstruation, because your basal temperature changes during the menstrual cycle.

Normal basal temperature is within the range of 36.55–36.78°C (97.8–98.2°F) . If your average temperature falls below or above this range you should seek the advice of a health practitioner.

This is a particularly useful test to do because it measures what you actually need to know: your production of

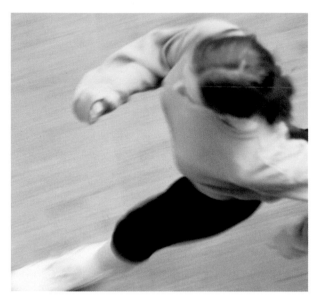

▲ *An increased pulse rate when exercising is normal. However, if you are suffering from a high pulse rate when just walking down the street or relaxing at home, this could prove to be a risk factor for osteoporosis.*

energy by way of body heat, rather than the amount of circulating hormones.

Pulse rate

An excessively rapid heartbeat when relaxed is a risk factor for osteoporosis. As you age you will want to pay attention to your heart and the state of your arteries, and this is not the place to go into all the relevant factors or to outline what you should do to have the healthiest heart possible. Nonetheless, many of the suggestions for changes in your diet and lifestyle outlined here will also benefit your heart. Such changes include the dietary recommendations that you should eat more fruit and vegetables and fewer processed foods, refined carbohydrates, white flour, sugar, saturated fats and so on. When you do make the suggested changes and improve the state of your heart and arteries you can be confident that you are also helping your bones. It should not really be surprising to find that a lifestyle that benefits one part of your body also benefits another, and, in fact, your whole body.

Weight factors associated with osteoporosis

- Being too thin.
- Losing more than 10 per cent of your body weight after the menopause unless it is done very gradually.

Homocysteine

Cysteine is a naturally occurring amino acid which is found in many proteins. Homocysteine, an altered form of cysteine, is now recognized as being harmful and indicative of the fact that the body is unable to reconvert it to cysteine and another related amino acid, methionine.

High levels of homocysteine in the blood are now thought to be a more accurate predictor of possible heart problems than high levels of cholesterol. There is also evidence that raised levels of homocysteine in the blood may be a contributory factor to osteoporosis.

This is discussed further, together with what to do about it if you have the problem, under folic acid and vitamin B (see page 40).

Vision

If you have poor depth perception you are at increased risk of developing osteoporosis. Like being tall, use this, if your depth perception is poor, as a prompt to put in place the various lifestyle changes that will help to lower your risk in other ways.

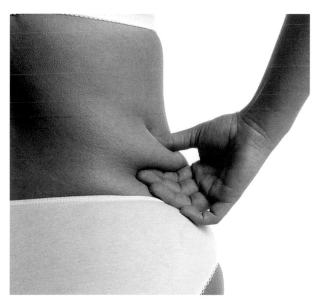

▲ *The good news for everyone is that being too slim can actually have negative effects; carrying around a small amount of extra weight can be beneficial to your bones.*

Lifestyle

You may be unable to do anything about your genes and hereditary factors predisposing you to bone weaknesses, but you can do much to change your lifestyle to improve the strength and density of your bones.

Weight

We hear so often that we should lose weight that it may come as a pleasant surprise to learn that it is possible to be too slim and that having a small amount of extra weight may be of some benefit. The evidence suggests that if you are slim or too thin you could run an increased risk of developing osteoporosis.

An overactive thyroid gland (see page 29), a known risk for osteoporosis, could be causing your lack of body weight. In addition, if you are too thin and do not have sufficient adipose tissue you will be less able to produce oestrogen from this source.

You should also bear in mind that exercise helps to prevent osteoporosis, particularly weight-bearing exercise that puts pressure on your bones (running or brisk walking, for example, is more effective than swimming). Carrying a slight amount of excess weight can be considered a form of weight-bearing exercise and may actually help to push calcium into your bones.

It is important to keep things in proportion. Note that the problems start if you are slim or too thin. Having a normal body weight for your height is excellent, it may even be helpful to be slightly overweight. It is not helpful to be considerably overweight. It is not good for your general health, and it does not play a part in the prevention of bone problems, because a significant (as distinct to a slight) excess of weight to carry around is going to put great pressure on your bones. It will also reduce your flexibility and agility and, probably, reduce your interest in taking up an exercise programme.

It is much better never to gain excess weight in the first place. However, if you have become overweight and want to lose some, the timing of any weight loss is important. Ideally, you should do it before the start of the menopause. Research suggests that after the menopause it is better to stay the weight you are than to go on a sudden weight-loss programme and lose more than 10 per cent of your body weight, which can double your risk of getting osteoporosis.

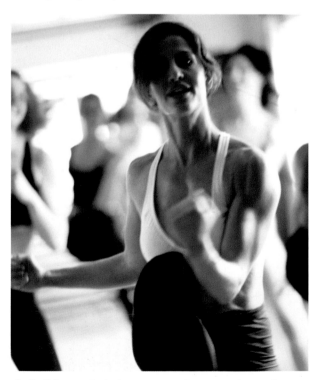

▲ *Building muscle tone goes a long way towards protecting your bones and body from accidents and fractures by helping to increase your balance and driving calcium into the bones.*

Height

It is not, of course, possible to do anything about your height, but it is interesting to find that the tall, willowy blonde (or brunette) may be at a disadvantage. Statistics show that tall women are more likely to develop osteoporosis than their shorter sisters. If you are tall you should pay additional attention to the things you can do to minimize your risk of developing osteoporosis.

Muscle tone and balance

Age and muscle tone may be good indicators of your risk of fracturing a bone (see page 13), and some exercises that may be helpful for muscle tone are described in Part 4. For the moment it is important to stress that you should do all you can to change those flabby muscles to taut ones because exercise:
• helps drive calcium into your bones
• will improve your overall control of your body
• may make you steadier on your feet and improve your balance
• will make you better able to move quickly to regain your balance if you do trip
• reduces the risk that you will fracture bones since you will be less likely to fall

Exercise

Lack of exercise is a significant risk factor in the development of osteoporosis. If you sit around and do nothing, calcium tends to leave your bones. If you run, calcium tends to enter your bones. The critical factor is that the exercise should be weight-bearing. The more you use your bones and make demands on them, the stronger they become.

Swimming is an excellent form of exercise, particularly for people with arthritis or other types of joint problem. However, it will do little to strengthen your bones because the water, rather than your bones, carries your weight. Run, if you can, or go for brisk walks. Do press-ups or push-ups, which apply weight to specific bones.

Being confined to bed is one of the best ways to encourage osteoporosis to develop. If you break a leg, for example, and, as a result, don't use it, you will slow down the repair processes. If, on the other hand, you apply gentle pressure to the bone you will encourage calcium back into it and thus accelerate the repair process. If you are concerned about this, consult with your health practitioner to establish just how much is a safe amount of pressure to apply. If you are confined to bed for any reason you should still exercise, and simply pressing your feet firmly against the end of the bed will help to drive some more calcium into the bones of your legs.

Alcohol

Alcohol is a socially acceptable drug. In spite of its widely recognized and well-publicized harmful side effects it is now a securely entrenched part of our lifestyle.

Heavy drinkers, however, lose many nutrients in urine because of the diuretic effect of alcohol. This includes important minerals and vitamins needed by your bones. Alcohol specifically increases the urinary loss of calcium, magnesium, copper, zinc and vitamin C and, at the same time, inhibits the absorption of calcium. In addition, when you drink alcohol food calories are replaced by alcohol calories, so there is a decreased intake of essential nutrients, including calcium and the other minerals needed by bones. The more alcohol you drink, the greater is this effect.

Among young men and women who had died suddenly it has been found that the bone density of young, heavy drinkers in particular was reduced to a level similar to that found in older, post-menopausal women. On the other hand, young non-drinkers and light drinkers had bone densities considered to be normal and healthy for their age. The bone density of chronic heavy drinkers may be reduced to between 90 and 60 per cent of a normal level for their age compared to teetotallers or light drinkers.

Calcium loss

Calcium that is found in urine is calcium that has already been absorbed and transported throughout the system. Any calcium lost in the faeces, in contrast, is calcium that has passed straight through the digestive system and has not been absorbed at all.

It does seem that an average alcohol intake equivalent to one drink a day does not cause problems. The ongoing Framingham study, which has been monitoring people for more than 40 years, seems to indicate that an average intake of a drink a day (but no more) is actually associated with greater bone density in post-menopausal woman.

Caffeine

Caffeine is found in tea, coffee, chocolate, cola drinks and other soft drinks. It is just one of the harmful compounds in those drinks, and although it is usually blamed for any harmful effects of the beverages, several other compounds also produce symptoms of toxicity. Coffee is no longer considered to be benign. Instead, it is recognized as having a number of deleterious effects, and although it is socially sanctioned it is a drug, with addictive, behaviour-modifying characteristics. In addition to the damage it can do in other ways – its effect on the adrenal glands, heart and nervous system, for example – it can also affect your bones.

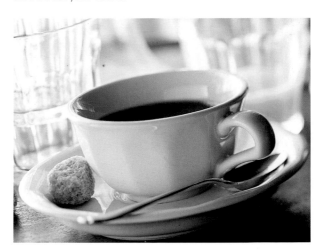

▲ Coffee can have damaging effects not only on your bones, but also on your adrenal glands, heart and nervous system.

Many women take oestrogen when they are going through or have passed the menopause in order to stop the hot flushes and, ironically, to maintain calcium levels. Yet if you are taking oestrogen and also drinking coffee, there will be an increased loss of calcium in urine after each cup of coffee. As a result, much of the hoped-for beneficial effect of the oestrogen will be lost.

It has been found that male volunteers who drank three cups of coffee a day had an increased urinary loss of both calcium and magnesium. Even young women, those in their 30s, can be adversely affected by coffee. You may think that an intake of one or two cups a day is safe and acceptable, yet that amount has been shown to result in a daily urinary loss of over 20mg of calcium. For each extra cup of coffee drunk, the loss of calcium was increased by 6mg. The situation is worsened because people who drink several cups of coffee a day also tend to eat a more highly processed and low-calcium diet.

Bear in mind that you only have to lose 40mg of calcium a day to then lose between 1 and 1.5 per cent of your bone mass each year, particularly if you are post-menopausal.

It is known that a high intake of caffeine, whether from coffee, cola drinks, tea, chocolate or any other source, is associated with an increased frequency of bone fractures and an increased incidence of osteoporosis, probably caused by the increasing urinary loss of both calcium and magnesium. If you drink five or more cups of coffee a day, your risk of getting osteoporosis is increased almost threefold. Even if you drink only an average of two cups a day, over a period of years, your risk is increased.

Although caffeine is an addictive and behaviour-modifying drug it is easier to give up than a hard drug. You may have withdrawal headaches for a few days, but after that there are rarely any symptoms. You then have to work on changing your behaviour patterns.

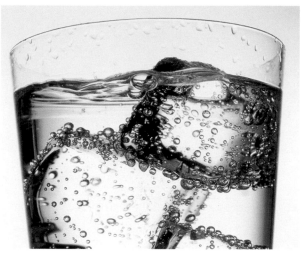

▲ *Many fizzy drinks contain sugar, artificial flavourings and too much phosphorus, with caffeine added to increase their appeal.*

You can give up coffee without causing a significant disruption to your social life. There are many alternatives to coffee, including dandelion root coffee, which has the advantage that is particularly good for your liver (see page 23 for a discussion of liver's role in the metabolism of vitamin D and calcium). Tea can be replaced by a variety of herb teas. Many restaurants now offer herbal teas. Cola drinks can be replaced by fruit juice or mineral water. All these are healthier alternatives to their caffeine-laden counterparts, not only because they don't contain caffeine and don't contribute to osteoporosis, but also because they offer other health benefits as well.

Carbonated drinks

Soft, fizzy drinks are made from sugar, water, flavourings and colouring agents. There may or may not be some fruit juice in them. They generally also contain a variety of other chemicals, including, in many cases, caffeine (see above). In fact, it is often the caffeine that gives them their 'kick' and their appeal. When a leading soft drink manufacturer decided to remove the caffeine from one of its bestselling products for health reasons it found its sales falling to a level that it could not sustain. So it put the caffeine back, and the popularity of the drink gradually rose back to the earlier levels.

Caffeine is not the only problem with these soft drinks. To make them fizz, chemicals are added that produce carbon dioxide. Unfortunately, these chemicals make the drinks taste acidic and unpleasant. To overcome this problem phosphate compounds are added to 'buffer' the solution. In practice, this means that they 'mop up' the acid to make the drink neutral and pleasant to taste.

Remember what was said about phosphorus earlier (see page 21). To maintain the strength of your bones you should consume equal amounts of calcium and phosphorus. There is little or no calcium in soft drinks, but there is a lot of phosphorus. A high intake of phosphates can lead to an increased loss of calcium in your urine and thus to weaker bones.

Smoking

The importance of oestrogen to strong bones is widely recognized, so it seems unwise to do anything to jeopardize the levels of this hormone in your body. Yet this is just what smoking does. In post-menopausal women it

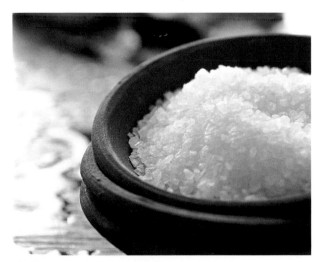

▲ *Try to avoid adding salt to your food as it can affect your bones by increasing the loss of calcium in urine.*

has been shown that smoking can reduce the oestrogen level by as much as 50 per cent.

As a result, people who smoke, particularly post-menopausal women, can expect to have a significantly higher incidence of osteoporosis than their non-smoking counterparts. Cigarette smoking also depletes the body of ascorbic acid and exposes it to a number of toxins, such as cadmium and lead, which directly damage bone and interfere with calcium absorption.

Salt

In addition to the other well-known adverse affects of too much salt on your body, it affects bones by increasing the loss of calcium in urine. This is another good reason for omitting salt from your diet and learning to appreciate the subtle flavours of the foods themselves.

Medicines

Many of the drugs taken for medical reasons have an adverse effect on bones. The tranquillizer benzodiazepine, for example, has been shown to increase the risks of bone fractures by up to 70 per cent, and many types of sleeping pills can have a similar effect.

Steroid medications are particularly harmful and have a significant adverse effects on bones.

• They reduce the activity of the osteoblasts, the bone-building cells.
• They make existing osteoblasts more responsive to parathyroid hormone and vitamin D, which, in turn, activate the osteoclasts that break down bones.
• They slow down the synthesis of collagen, which leads to faulty bone cells.
• They inhibit calcium absorption from the intestine.

If you are taking, or have taken, these drugs you should make particular efforts to do all you can to build up your bones and prevent further development of osteoporosis.

What Bones Need

Your bones need many nutrients, vitamins and minerals and a wide range of other compounds, and these are found in fruits, vegetables and other foods. So the first step, when you are considering the health of your bones, is to think about your diet.

Don't stop thinking there. Consider what supplements you could take to improve still further on the dietary changes you have made. Do not, however, fall into the trap of thinking that you can simply take a handful of supplements and use them as an excuse to eat whatever junk foods you like: it is important that you also make the beneficial changes to your diet that are recommended on pages 46–57.

In the remainder of this chapter we will look at the individual nutrients your bones need so that you can begin to alter your diet and start planning a supplement programme.

Minerals

When they think about their bones, most people think of calcium, and this is, of course, important, but many other minerals are involved, and without these (in the proper proportions) all the calcium in the world will not stop the development of osteoporosis. In fact, calcium on its own could even do harm.

Calcium

Calcium is a major component of the mineral structure of your bones, so clearly it is important to make sure you get an adequate amount. You lose some calcium every day, mainly in urine, and it is vital that this amount is replaced. If you are pregnant you will need more calcium for the formation of the extra bones you are making (see page 28). If you don't take in sufficient calcium your bones will gradually be depleted of it, and osteoporosis will develop. A daily dose of 1,000mg is generally recommended, with an increase to 1,500mg close to and after the menopause.

Reducing calcium loss

Many factors increase the body's loss of calcium in urine. These include the following, which should be reduced or avoided:
- a high intake of phosphorus or a phosphorus-rich diet
- a high-protein intake; keep to your daily requirement and don't eat more
- caffeine, found in tea and coffee; even two or three cups a day can be significant
- salt
- sugar
- magnesium deficiency

Substances that reduce urinary loss of calcium:
- boron
- oestrogen
- vitamin K

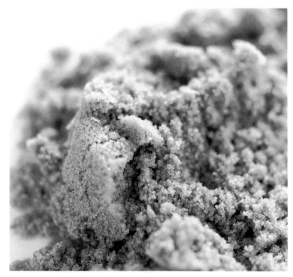

▲ *Using too much sugar in your diet will actually deplete your body of calcium resulting in an increased risk of developing osteoporosis.*

Osteoporosis is a common problem among the elderly, but you should be aware that even women as young as 20 years old can develop weakened bones when their diet is inadequate. Clearly, osteoporosis can start early on in life. No matter what your age, it is important that you improve your diet and consider the possible need for supplements. Check that you are eating a diet that supplies a large amount of calcium. If not, it is time to make some positive changes.

Should you be taking supplements, and, if so, what sort? In general it seems that there is 30–40 per cent absorption of the calcium taken as calcium carbonate, calcium acetate or calcium gluconate. This compares with a figure of about 30 per cent absorption of calcium from milk. Calcium ascorbate is another useful supplement and is easily absorbed. It is approximately 10 per cent calcium and 90 per cent vitamin C, so you are getting the benefit of both nutrients. Calcium citrate-malate is another effective form, as is hydroxyapatite, the mineral from which bone is made (see page 17).

Stomach acid helps digestion and absorption in general and that includes the digestion and absorption of calcium-rich foods and supplements. Most people produce less stomach acid as they get older, and because calcium absorption is more difficult when stomach acid levels are low, it might be sensible to take a supplement with additional hydrochloric acid and digestive enzymes to further aid calcium absorption.

Phosphorus

As we have seen (page 21), calcium is partnered by phosphorus in bones, and the ideal diet would provide them in equal amounts. Unfortunately, the foods commonly eaten in the Western diet contain a considerable excess of phosphorus over calcium.

The average Western diet has a ratio of calcium to phosphorus that varies between 1:2 and 1:4, which means that it has two to four times as much phosphorus as calcium. Even when the ratio is 1:2 bone reabsorption occurs and osteoporosis can develop, regardless of the total amount of calcium ingested. Other studies suggest that an even lower excess of phosphorus over calcium can be just as harmful and that even if the calcium to phosphorus ratio is 1:1.25 (instead of the ideal 1:1) attempts to treat osteoporosis may be unsuccessful unless the phosphorus intake is reduced.

One of the disadvantages of a high phosphorus intake is its effect on parathyroid hormone. Phosphorus can increase calcium loss from bones by causing nutritional hyperparathyroidism, which pulls calcium from bones. The intake of high levels of phosphorus can also lead to reduced vitamin D activity and hence reduced absorption of calcium from the digestive system.

In general, the foods rich in phosphorus are the acid-forming foods (see page 54). These foods are the ones that leave an acid residue in your body when they have been metabolized, and include meat, protein-rich foods in general and grains. In the interests of preventing osteoporosis you should reduce your intake of these foods to the minimum that will provide adequate amounts of protein. Many meats and other acid-forming foods contain as much as 20–30 parts of phosphorus for each part of calcium. Most fruits and vegetables, even the seemingly acid ones, leave an alkaline residue in the body and have a much better balance of calcium and phosphorus; these should make up a large part of your diet.

It can't be said too often: eat vegetables, lots of them, and then some more. Whenever you want a snack think about vegetables and fruit and not about acid-forming foods and try to make vegetables a part of your daily life.

As we have noted (see page 34), carbonated soft drinks contain a significant amount of phosphate and little or no calcium and so should be avoided.

Importance of magnesium

A long-term deficiency of magnesium:
• is associated with reduced production of parathyroid hormone and reduced absorption of both dietary and supplementary calcium
• reduces the kidneys' response to parathyroid hormone because the mechanism regulating the amount of calcium lost in urine becomes less effective
• is associated with a reduction in the efficiency of vitamin D, which can reduce calcium absorption.

Magnesium
Approximately 70 per cent of the body's magnesium is stored in the bones, where it replaces some of the calcium (to which it is structurally similar) and where it has a subtle, but important, influence on bone structure. Magnesium also has an effect on the activity of parathyroid hormone.

People with osteoporosis often have a deficiency of magnesium, which may be one of the contributing factors. It is particularly important to bear this in mind because many of the medications prescribed for osteoporosis contain calcium and vitamin D but either no, or very little, magnesium, even though it may be needed even more urgently than calcium by some people.

Manganese
Small amounts of manganese (which should not be confused with magnesium) are found in bones. This trace mineral is also important for the body's softer, connective tissues, which include the covering tissue around the bones themselves and the tendons, ligaments and cartilage. Many knee problems could be solved or prevented if a developing manganese deficiency had been identified and corrected in time.Making sure that you get an adequate intake of this element may help to prevent many of the joint problems that hinder your ability to do the exercises that, in turn, are important for maintaining bone strength.

It is probable that you are lacking manganese if:
• your knees click or creak, especially when you squat
• you have 'hang nails' (the spiky bits of tough skin that can stick up along the sides of your fingernails)
• you get motion sick, such as when reading in the back seat of a car
• your 'blind' balance is poor – you can't stand on one leg with your eyes closed as well as you can with your eyes open
• you have been taking a zinc supplement without added manganese

Zinc
The trace element zinc is one of the micro-nutrients that occupy spaces within the hydroxyapatite crystalline structure. Elderly people with osteoporosis often have below-normal levels of zinc.

Zinc is important to the bones both functionally and structurally. It is needed for building cartilage, but also for breaking down old and unwanted cartilage and for preventing the build-up of fibrous tissue after accidents and trauma. It is needed for the formation of DNA and RNA, by means of which your cells are programmed.

Copper
The element copper plays a role in bone metabolism. If your drinking water has passed through copper piping you are unlikely to be lacking in copper, but if your water supply passes through non-copper pipes you may need a copper supplement.

You can determine the amount of copper present in your body by measuring the amount present in a sample of hair. A qualified naturopath can calculate this for you.

Some people find that copper bracelets help or ease their problems with arthritis. If this is the case it is probably because they are deficient in copper, and the amount absorbed through the skin is sufficient to make good all or some of the deficiency.

Silica

Silica is necessary for bone formation, and occurs where there is active bone growth. It is important in determining the rate at which the bone is mineralized. Studies on animals have shown that silica deficiency can be associated with abnormal skeletal development, producing bones that are thinner, less flexible and contain less collagen than normal. If your fingernails are weak or are liable to break easily you could be short of silica. Good sources of silica are oat bran, the herb equisetum (horsetail) and the tissue salt, silicea.

Boron

Boron interacts with many mineral nutrients and has a beneficial effect on the treatment and prevention of both osteoporosis and arthritis. It reduces the amounts of calcium and magnesium that are lost in urine. It can compensate for a lack of vitamin D, help to increase the effect of the vitamin D that is available, and may improve the synthesis of vitamin D.

In the body boron is found in the highest concentrations in bones that are actively growing or are being calcified, and it is now thought that boron is needed for optimal bone formation and strength.

The highest amounts of boron can be found in vegetables, fruits, beans and nuts. It is also found in kelp and some seaweeds. An intake of 4–6mg a day seems to give beneficial results. Extremely high doses can be harmful, but even a dose rate of up to 100mg a day seems to produce no obvious side effects in humans. This may be because boron does not accumulate in the body and is readily lost in urine.

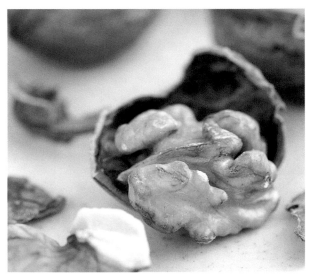

▲ *Nuts are an excellent source of boron in the diet, and this mineral is needed as a deterrent for osteoporosis and arthritis.*

An additional benefit of taking boron is that it is known to improve brain function, enhancing concentration, perception and memory, and to improve manual dexterity and eye-to-hand coordination.

Fluoride

Fluoride has been found to be helpful in preventing childhood dental caries, though there can be disadvantages when it is used to excess. Following from this it has been suggested that it could also help to prevent osteoporosis, particularly if taken as Calc. Fluor., which is readily available in most health foods shops.

Vitamins

All the different types of tissue in your body need all the different vitamins and your bones are no exception. The cells of your bones, for example, need vitamins B1, B2, B3, B5, biotin and others, which are involved in the production of energy, and vitamin E, which is an important anti-oxidant. Some vitamins are particularly important for your bones, and these are discussed on the following pages.

Vitamin A

Vitamin A (retinol) stimulates the production of progesterone, the hormone that is now thought to be more useful than oestrogen in the prevention of osteoporosis. You can get it from eggs and meats, especially liver. Carotenes, the precursors of vitamin A, are available from bright orange, red or green plant foods, such as carrots, beetroot and leafy green vegetables.

Folic acid and vitamins B6 and B12

A chemical known as homocysteine is rapidly becoming recognized as a harmful compound that is implicated in increased risks of heart disease (see page 31). It can also damage your bones and collagen. Homocysteine levels can be kept low by making sure that you have adequate amounts of vitamins B6 (pyridoxine) and B12 (cyanocobalamin) and of betaine (an alkaloid present in sugar beet and other vegetables). Even when the levels of these vitamins have been reported as normal in the blood, homocysteine levels have fallen when people took a supplement with as much as 5000mcg folic acid. This is a safe dose but should always be taken in combination with some vitamin B12. Otherwise the folic acid can mask a possible B12 deficiency.

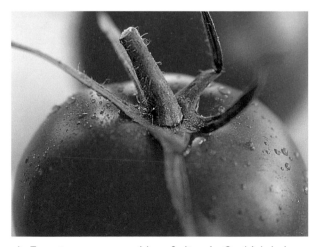

▲ *Tomatoes are a provider of vitamin C which helps to give the bones their strength by holding the collagen fibres together.*

Vitamin C

Vitamin C (ascorbic acid) plays so many roles in the body that it is not surprising to find it active in the bones. It is essential for the formation of collagen and for holding the collagen fibres together, thus contributing to their strength and resilience. The disease most often associated with vitamin C deficiency is scurvy, and the main symptoms of the disease – loose teeth, bleeding gums, painful joints and so on – involve the breakdown of the connective collagen tissues.

Vitamin C also increases the production of progesterone. When vitamin C occurs in foods it is generally found in combination with bioflavonoids, some of which, known as OPCs, have been shown to make vitamin C nearly 11 times more effective than it would be alone. The best way to improve your intake of vitamin C is to eat foods that contain all these compounds, especially fruit, such as oranges and strawberries, and the fruits of other plants, such as tomatoes and sweet peppers. These nutrients are also found in the green leaves of a wide range of vegetables.

If you are taking a supplement look for one that contains vitamin C in calcium form (calcium ascorbate) in combination with bioflavonoids.

Vitamin D

Vitamin D works with parathyroid hormone to aid in the absorption of calcium from the intestinal tract and the maintenance of normal levels of blood calcium. In both the prevention and treatment of osteoporosis, giving vitamin D in conjunction with calcium is much more effective than giving calcium on its own.

Remember that it is not just a simple matter of consuming vitamin D or of making it while your skin is exposed to the sun. Before it can do its job it must be converted to 25HCC in the liver, and to 1:25DHCC in the kidneys, processes that become less efficient with age. In some people the problem has advanced to a stage where the final active form, 1:25 DHCC, is not produced. This should be discussed with your doctor. For most people, however, ensuring an adequate intake of the vitamin, a sensible amount of exposure to the sun and taking care to look after your kidneys and liver will make a significant difference to calcium absorption.

Vitamin K

Vitamin K used to be regarded as a 'one-job' vitamin and known as the clotting factor. We now know that it will not make blood clot; instead, it facilitates the process when all the other triggers are in place. Taking it cannot, of itself, cause blood clots to form.

The vitamin does both this and the other jobs it performs by working with calcium, encouraging calcium deposition in the bones and discouraging its deposition where it is not wanted, such as in the artery walls.

Many post-menopausal women stop losing calcium in urine when they take vitamin K, which does not have the unwanted side effects of oestrogen. Taking it in combination with ipriflavone (see page 61) works well.

Not only does Vitamin K help prevent heart disease and strokes and stop the development of osteoporosis, it also protects you from cancer, keeps the brain alert, reduces the incidence of Alzheimer's disease and the risk of high blood pressure and helps to keep you young. It surely deserves more attention than it has been getting.

Most problems associated with vitamin K deficiency are linked to advancing age. They include high blood pressure, heart attacks, strokes, osteoporosis and senility. Making sure that your diet includes a high intake of this vitamin is an important way of staying young and increasing your chances of avoiding, or certainly postponing, many of the problems that come with age, including osteoporosis.

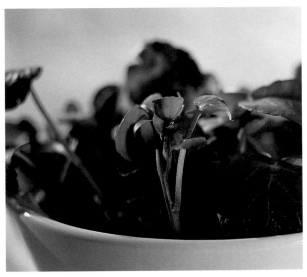

▲ *Watercress and leafy green vegetables are excellent sources of vitamin K which is very important in the fight against osteoporosis as, among other things, it supplies calcium and other minerals.*

Vitamin K is yet another reason why you should eat your greens, particularly leafy green vegetables, broccoli and cauliflower. As with so many of the important nutrients, the richest sources of this vitamin are vegetables.

Because it is fat-soluble, vitamin K should be eaten or taken with some form of fat. If your fat absorption is faulty you may be consuming this vitamin but not absorbing it, and this can become increasingly likely as you get older and your liver and gall bladder start to function less well.

Vitamin K2, another form of the vitamin, is produced by bacteria and other micro-organisms in your digestive tract. For most healthy people this is a major source of vitamin K, so it is important to make sure your intestinal tract is healthy. Unlike other fat-soluble vitamins, vitamin K is not stored in the body and so is less likely to be toxic in high doses. Although 10mg a day is a commonly recommended dose, amounts up to 50mg a day have been used without adverse effects.

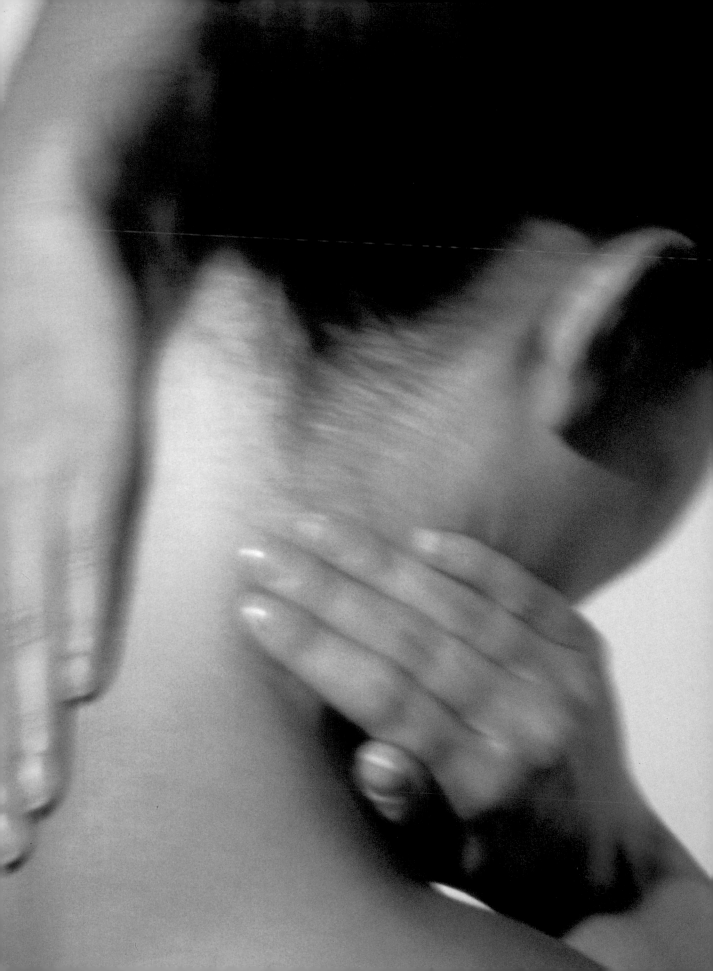

Treatment 2

Clearly prevention is better than cure. Equally clearly, the best time to practise prevention is when you are young. However, few young people consider the health problems that they could develop in older age, and osteoporosis is just such a problem. Unless you are exceptional, if you are reading this you are probably already in or approaching middle age and are already facing the possibility of developing, or having started to develop, osteoporosis.

Medical Intervention

Prescription drugs

If you have osteoporosis you may be prescribed some of the drugs that have been suggested for treatment. They can generally be divided into two types.

1 Those aimed at preventing the resorption or breakdown of bones may decrease the activity of the osteoclasts (see page 10) or decrease the activity of parathyroid hormones on the bones, thus preventing the removal of calcium from the bones as well as preventing bone breakdown.

2 Those aimed at increasing the activity of the osteoblasts (see page 10) may enhance the effect of calcitonin and increase the uptake of calcium from the blood by the bones, thus promoting bone-building.

The two processes are, however, closely linked together, and if you alter one it is probable that you will also affect the other. This means that many of the drugs that help to prevent bone reabsorption by the osteoclasts (good) also reduce the activity of the osteoblasts (bad). This is particularly true when they are used on a long-term basis.

The first group of drugs described above includes oestrogen (hormone), calcium, bisphosphonates and calcitonin (hormone). The second group includes sodium fluoride, anabolic fragments of parathyroid hormone and insulin-like growth factor.

Unfortunately, these drugs have other adverse effects. For example, sodium fluoride increases bone density, but it also changes the crystalline structure of the bones and actually makes them more fragile. Therefore it is often better to adopt a naturopathic approach to treatment.

Naturopathy

In the naturopathic treatment of most health problems there are generally several clearly defined steps to take, although the precise details may vary from one practitioner to another.

- Make appropriate lifestyle changes, such as exercising and relaxing.
- Correct your diet to make sure that it contains the maximum amounts possible of all the necessary nutrients and to eliminate all kinds of harmful foods, substances and practices.
- Add special foods and nutritional herbs, which can generally be added to your diet and included in the various dishes you prepare.
- Add supplements of specific nutrients as appropriate.
- Take specific remedies, herbal or homoeopathic medicines.

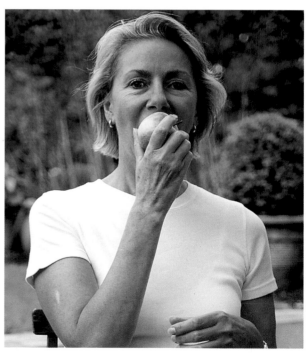

▲ *It is imperative that your diet includes the full range of nutrients needed by bones. This, combined with regular weight-bearing exercise, will increase your chances of deterring osteoporosis.*

Osteoporosis prevention plan

Osteoporosis in later life can best be prevented by a multi-step plan that includes:

○ paying attention to all the known risk factors

○ making any lifestyle changes that are indicated

○ changing your diet so that it provides the maximum amount of the necessary nutrients and minimizes your intake of harmful factors

○ including in your diet some less common foods that may be helpful, such as soya-based foods and seaweeds

○ ensuring an adequate intake of calcium supplements as appropriate

○ having an adequate intake of all the other nutrients needed by the bones and taking the appropriate supplements as necessary

○ doing moderate amounts of physical weight-bearing exercise

○ if you are female and over the age of 40, taking oestrogen with progesterone to slow the rate of bone loss (although it is not clear whether this therapy is advisable or necessary for all menopausal women)

○ optimizing the function of all the other organs involved in normal bone metabolism, including the liver, kidneys, parathyroid gland, thyroid gland, adrenal glands and digestive system

What you eat is crucially important to your health and general wellbeing, and it is amazing that medicine does not give diet the serious attention it deserves or take a more thorough and careful approach to assessing the effect it has on our health. No one would say that the type of petrol you put in your car is unimportant, yet a car is a simple machine compared to the complexities of the human body. There may be some rational explanation for how and why this happened in the past, but there is no excuse, given our knowledge of nutrition and human biochemistry, for continuing with this attitude today.

Nutrition and the medical profession

Multinational drug companies make drugs and medications that are patented and make the companies wealthy. Vitamins, minerals and raw foods cannot be patented. The drug companies have the advertising power, the sales forces, the resources to produce multiple technical brochures, to run seminars and more. For the busy doctor, it is all too easy to accept the latest information on the latest drug. Furthermore, because doctors do not generally study nutrition in medical school, learning about it when they are practising so that they can offer constructive and detailed advice on diet is generally not even considered.

As a result, modern medicine has never fully embraced nutrition, even though the science, biochemistry and application of it are well researched and widely written up in the scientific literature. At best, if you are concerned about osteoporosis, your doctor will tell you to take more calcium and eat a well-balanced diet.

Overlooking the nutritional aspects of health care can cause untold harm. Even the concept of a 'well-balanced' diet, which your doctor may suggest you should adopt, is far from helpful, and it is worth taking a look at this as background to some of the suggestions that are made later in this chapter.

Diet

How our diet has evolved

To understand the effect of today's diet on your health it is worth paying attention to what humans have eaten as they evolved over millions of years. Consider the time span from the Cave Age until relatively recently, about 15,000 to 10,000 years ago. It consisted essentially of plant foods, fruits, vegetables and the flesh of wild animals. During this period our bodies and our diets co-evolved and co-adapted. Individuals for whom the available diet was most satisfactory survived and had the healthiest and most viable offspring – our own ancestors.

On this scale the past 10,000 years is a very short period and it is reasonable to assume that we have not evolved far away from this Cave-age diet and that basing our diet today on these same foods could be beneficial. This hypothesis is worth considering as is its relevance to the prevention of osteoporosis. If we find that many of the foods that help to prevent osteoporosis are also the ones that made up the majority of the Cave-age diet, this can help to reassure us that the suggested changes will be beneficial and not a harmful departure from what we now consider to be 'normal'.

In just the past few thousand years, a tiny fraction of our evolutionary history, major changes have been made to our diet. The past few decades have brought about even greater change. It is highly unlikely that we have had time to co-evolve and adapt to these changes. We may be able to tolerate these changes but there is no clear evidence that they are beneficial or any improvement on our previous Cave-age diet. Furthermore, because we now have the medical technology to keep people alive for longer we may be keeping alive those for whom the modern diet is definitely not the optimum one.

In other words it is possible that this Cave-age diet would still be a healthy diet, and possibly our healthiest diet. To assess this hypothesis, I have, in the past constructed a variety of diets based on several

The Cave-age diet

The Cave-age diet can be broken down as follows:
- approximately 75–80 per cent of the diet was fruit and vegetable
- 20 per cent of the diet was flesh – animal, bird or fish
- some nuts and seeds
- fresh herbs

No, or limited amounts of:
- dairy products
- grains (wheat, barley, oats, rye, rice etc)
- alcohol
- sugar, only honey when they could find it – it was not a regular part of their diet

different versions of the so-called 'well-balanced diet', whether it be based on four, six or seven food groups, and have compared the nutrient content of these with a number of versions of the Cave-age diet, as indicated above.

It turns out that none of the textbook 'well-balanced diets' actually provide 100 per cent of all the vitamins and minerals you need. It is also clear that these diets are much better than the diets of most people today. Certainly they are much better than the diets of almost every patient I have seen in my 25 years in practice. Furthermore, the various Cave-age diets were very much better, in terms of overall nutritional status, than any of the 'well-balanced diets'.

You may be wondering about the place of grains, of bread, pasta and rice in the diet. You may be wondering about milk and dairy products that are supposed to be such a good source of calcium. You may even be wondering about butter and oils, about sugar, sweets and chocolates, thinking that surely some of them at least, might also be acceptable.

We will be addressing these topics later on. However while we are looking at this in a historical context it is worth pointing out that none of these foods were available to our Cave-age ancestors.

The twentieth-century diet

Whole grains

The grains we know today, with their dense heads of seeds have been selectively bred over the past few thousand years. To do this people had to stop being nomadic and live in fixed settlements. Only then could they plant seeds, nurture the plants and harvest the results. Nomads would have been unlikely to raise grasses for long enough to develop the dense seedheads we know today, because even if they had planted them they would not have been around to tend them or, later, to harvest them. As nomads, when the weather got cold and food got scarce, our forebears would have moved to a warmer region. It was only once they settled down and became farmers and had to grow and eat food that could be stored through the cold months that grains became an important part of the diet.

Milk

A similar logic can be applied to our consumption of dairy products. Wild animals do not stand around waiting to be milked, so until they were tamed and people became settled farmers it is unlikely that dairy products were consumed, certainly in any quantity. There are, of course, some nomadic tribes that take their camels with them and milk them as needed, but this is the exception and a relatively recent development.

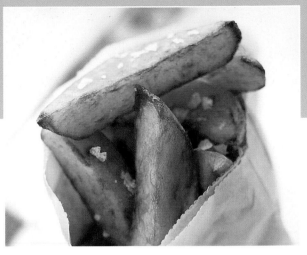

▲ *Change your diet to include more fruit and vegetables and cut out processed foods, such as chips, to give your body a fighting chance against osteoporosis.*

Allergenic foods

It is also worth pointing out that the top ten most common food allergens includes many of these recently introduced foods: grains, wheat, corn, rice, malt, rye, and dairy products. Clearly our 21st-century bodies have not yet adapted to these 'new' foods.

Processed foods

As for chocolate, sweets, sugar and all the processed foods of modern life, they have been introduced into our diet in just the last few decades. A lot has been said against their nutritional quality and effect on the body. There is very little if anything to say in their favour.

I am not suggesting that you should return to a pure Cave-age diet, even though the evidence suggests that this would be healthy. You live in the real world and this includes being able to socialize and to eat in restaurants. Becoming a recluse and never eating with friends or refusing to eat out because of a strict diet may have adverse emotional and social consequences that outweigh the health benefits. I am suggesting, however, that you assess the following dietary suggestions against this background. I think you will see that, in general and, wherever possible, you should consider the Cave-age diet as an ideal to be worked towards. I am also suggesting that you can move a long way from your present diet without restricting other aspects of your life.

Milk in the Cave-age diet?

People have been drinking milk only relatively recently in their evolution, but, as our forebears began to settle down, to farm animals and to use the spare milk that was available after the young had been weaned, they would almost certainly have drunk it whole – that is, with the fat included as we do today.

Protein

There are three major types of macronutrients: proteins, fats and carbohydrates. Everyone needs a certain amount of protein in their diet every day. Each day, even when you are completely healthy, some of your muscles (protein) and essential organs (protein) are broken down. In addition, some of the protein in your bones is lost. The proteins are broken into their constituent amino acids. Their carbon and hydrogen are converted into carbon dioxide and water respectively, and their nitrogen is converted into ammonia, which is lost in urine. These protein tissues have to be replaced by new tissue, which means that you need fresh protein to replace the old, and this new protein can come only from your diet.

You need protein so that your body can repair old and damaged tissues. If you cut yourself, you need protein for new tissue growth; if there is bleeding or if you suffer a burn you need new protein to replace those in the body fluids and tissue that are lost. You need protein to replace the cells lining your digestive tract and lungs and the cells of your skin, some of which are lost every day. Your body also needs protein to make a range of compounds, including:
• neurotransmitters – molecules that pass messages between nerves and muscles throughout your body and between the various nerve cells in the brain
• hormones – the messenger molecules that pass around your body in your blood and that act on distant tissues, triggering them into a variety of actions (some of these hormones are protein-based, the rest are steroid-based)
• enzymes – the catalysts that are needed to facilitate most of the chemical reactions that occur in the body

If you do not eat sufficient protein these vital neurotransmitters, hormones and enzymes will be unable to function properly. If, however, you eat more protein than you need for these and related purposes, the extra protein has to be used up, and the body turns spare protein into energy. This is not an efficient process, and it

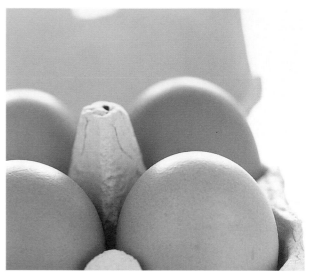

▲ *Eggs are an excellent source of protein in a well-balanced diet. Protein is needed to help the body repair damaged tissues.*

puts an unnecessary strain on your liver and kidneys, which have to process the extra nitrogen that proteins contain. In addition, the activity of breaking down the proteins and releasing their energy uses up about 30 per cent of the energy that they provide. The comparable figure for fats and carbohydrates is only 5 per cent.

There is also evidence that a high intake of protein leads to increased calcium loss in the urine, calcium that has

Too much protein

Eating more protein than you need:
◦ is an inefficient way of producing energy
◦ is an expensive way of producing energy because protein-rich foods usually cost more than other food types
◦ is a strain on your liver and kidneys
◦ causes increased calcium loss from your bones and body

come from the bones. People who eat an excessively high-protein diet have been found to be at increased risk of osteoporosis and to suffer from more fractures, especially of the hips. It is, therefore, important to determine approximately how much protein you need and to aim to include only about that amount in your diet on a daily basis.

In addition to the question of how much protein you should eat, there are considerations about its quality. Protein consists of approximately 20 different types of amino acid, of which half cannot be made in your body and must be provided by the diet. You can create the other ten for yourself by rearranging some of the first ten and you can, of course, get them from your diet.

To measure the quality of proteins the term 'net protein utilization' (NPU) is used. If the NPU is 100 the amino acids are present in exactly the right proportions, and you can use all the protein you consume for building your own protein. If it is zero at least one of the important amino acids is totally absent. In practice, all foods that contain protein, whether they are derived from animals or plants, have an NPU between these two extremes – a point that is often misunderstood. The only exception is gelatine, an animal protein, which has an NPU of zero.

Aiming for a high NPU allows you to make the most efficient use of the protein you eat. This is most easily achieved by eating animal proteins, particularly eggs and fish, which have a relatively high NPU, and slightly less efficiently by eating vegetable proteins, although some plant foods, such as rice and soya beans, have an NPU close to that of meat.

As a guide to working out how much protein you need, you should aim for approximately 0.8g of protein per kilogram (2.2lb) of body weight. This is an average figure and takes into account the differing NPUs of various foods and the fact that some of the protein will probably come from animal sources and some from vegetable sources, such as grains, beans and nuts.

Protein in the Cave-age diet?

The Cave-age diet contained protein in generous amounts when there had been a kill, but at other times it probably consisted mainly of fruits and vegetables.

Protein requirements

A man weighing 73kg (161lb) would need about 58g (2oz), and a woman weighing 57kg (126lb) would need about 45g(1½oz). The following table shows how much of each type of food you would need to eat to get the amount of protein you require. In practice you would eat some of several of these foods, but the information will allow you to work out your protein intake.

Food type	Average protein content (%)	Amount of food needed to give 45g (1½oz)	Amount of food needed to give 58g (2oz)
Most meats	22.5	200g (7oz)	260g (9z)
Eggs	12	375g (13oz)	480g (17oz)
Hard cheese	25	180g (6⅓oz)	232g (8oz)
Nuts & seeds	22.5	200g (7oz)	260g (9oz)
Dried beans	22.5	200g (7oz)	260g (9oz)
Grains	10.5	430g (15oz)	552g (1lb 3oz)

Types of protein

Once you have decided how much protein you need, you should find out which type of protein is the best for your bones – animal or plant.

As long as they get sufficient protein, vegetarians may have an advantage over meat-eaters. They have been found to have better bones, with a higher bone density, than people who eat a lot of the meat-based foods produced by modern agricultural methods. Modern farmed animals stand around in the fields all day and get fat. Not only is the flesh fattier, but the fat is also more saturated. We have already seen that ingesting more protein than is needed leads to increased calcium loss in urine. Some evidence suggests that plant protein leads to less calcium loss than animal protein and to avoid osteoporosis, you would be wise to adopt a vegetarian diet.

However, there are also suggestions that it is the other aspects of their diets that people change when they

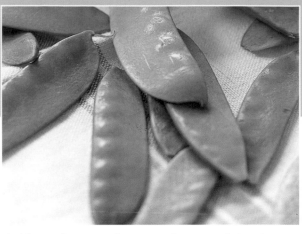

▲ *Vegetarians may have an advantage. It has been found that they have a higher bone density than people who regularly eat meat.*

decide to become vegetarian that may be important. For example, in general vegetarians are often less inclined to eat junk food and tend to take a greater interest in health foods than meat-eaters. The calcium to phosphorus and the calcium to magnesium ratios of their food are different, altering the whole nature of their diets.

Numerous analyses of diets have shown that people who eat a lot of meat often also eat a lot of fat, starches and sugar. Many meat-eaters have cereals or toast for breakfast, a meat, fish or cheese sandwich for lunch and a main meal of meat and some vegetables or pasta; they also eat sugary snacks, such as biscuits or chocolate. This is an acid-residue diet, high in protein but low in calcium, even if yogurt and cheese are included, and it is likely to lead to an increased risk of osteoporosis.

People who choose a vegetarian diet, with or without eggs and dairy products, generally focus on fruits and vegetables, from which they get more of the minerals they need for their bones and in a better balance (see page 54).

Fat

For many years now there has been a near-hysterical insistence that we should reduce the amount of fat in our diets to negligible proportions. A high-fat diet, it has been claimed, will lead to heart disease, cancer and strokes; a low-fat diet will lead to better health and greater longevity. Other people have claimed, however, that this is not so and that the real dietary culprits,

Fat in the Cave-age diet?

The Cave-age diet contained the fats found in meat and in nuts and seeds. The fats in the flesh of wild animals is also less saturated than that of domesticated farm animals. Wild animals, such as those caught by our early ancestors, lead a more active life than the cows and sheep kept on farms today. As a result, they carried little spare weight and a minimum of fat. Even the meat itself, the lean protein, contained much less fat marbled through it. Cutting off the visible fat is consistent with achieving this diet. Cavemen obviously did not eat margarine or the processed fats that are available today. They did not eat chips, crisps or high-fat pastries, nor did they eat over-heated fats.

causing many of our modern degenerative diseases, are the refined carbohydrates – that is, products made with white flour and laden with sugar – while fats have an important role to play in the diet.

Whether fat is bad for you largely depends on what type of fat you eat. Some animal fat is acceptable as long as it can be kept to a minimum. You can do this simply by removing the visible fat from meat and poultry, by using olive oil for cooking and making salad dressings and by making sure that you have a good supply of fish oils, either by eating oily fish or by taking supplements.

Types of fat

It is important to avoid margarine, hydrogenated fats and various other processed fats, which can cause a variety of problems. Some of the fats in margarine, for instance, have been converted from the healthy cis-form to the unhealthy trans-form, which can actually increase your level of cholesterol. This is true even though advertising claims the contrary. Avoid overcooked fats, such as those found in fried foods, crisps, roasted nuts and the like. The higher the temperature to which fats are heated the greater is the production of carcinogenic compounds. Once you get above the temperature at which you can sauté onions without them going brown, the rate of production of these compounds increases exponentially. Some interesting information is available about the fats in dairy food. If you mention the word osteoporosis to many people, they assume that they should be consuming more dairy foods by drinking more milk and eating more cheese and yogurt, in the belief that this is the best way to provide their body with the calcium it needs. (This is largely a fallacy, which we will be discussing later; see page 55.) At the same time people usually also feel that they should avoid consuming animal fats or a high-fat diet and so they choose skimmed milk, low-fat yogurt and low-fat cheeses. There is, however, a problem with this.

Fats are made up of fatty acids. Some of these are long, thin molecules (known as long-chain fatty acids); others are much shorter (short-chain fatty acids). Most of the fats from both animal and plant sources are made of long-chain fatty acids. Milk fat is different, however: it contains a significant amount of short-chain fatty acids. It seems that we need short-chain fatty acids to optimize the absorption of the calcium in dairy products. Thus, if you are going to consume dairy products for the calcium they contain you should consume them intact, not after the important short-chain fatty acids have been removed. If you still feel you should reduce your fat intake and you want to eat dairy products, drink full cream milk but reduce your fat intake in some other aspect of your diet.

Carbohydrates

When they talk about carbohydrates, many people think about bread, pasta, rice, cakes, pastry, biscuits and porridge. In other words, they think of wheat, rye, rice, oats, barley and other grains, such as millet and spelt (a type of wheat), and pseudo-cereals, such as quinoa and amaranthus. Carbohydrates are, however, found in many other foods. Beans and lentils contain about as much carbohydrate as they do protein, and the major component of most fruits and vegetables is carbohydrates. The other important carbohydrate in most people's lives is sugar.

What role do these foods play in osteoporosis? Grains and sugars are generally acid-forming, and their consumption should be reduced. Increasing your intake of carbohydrates in the form of refined (grain) carbohydrates and sugars leads to increased urinary loss of calcium. Eating carbohydrates in the form of fruits and vegetables means that you are increasing your consumption of alkaline-residue foods, and this is to be encouraged.

Sugar and other sweeteners

Sugar was most definitely not one of the foods enjoyed by our ancient ancestors. They would have had small amounts of honey on the rare occasions they found and were able to take the honey stored by wild bees. Today, however, sugar is one of our cheapest foods and probably the one that does us the most harm. It provides absolutely nothing of benefit: it does not contain a single vitamin or mineral; it is devoid of body-building protein; and it contains no essential fatty acid. All it gives are 'empty' calories.

You will know that there is sugar in sweets and chocolate bars; in most desserts, cakes and biscuits and in ice cream and soft drinks. However, much of the sugar you eat is invisible and it is more than likely that you are unaware of it. Sugar is hidden in most pre-packaged and processed foods, and it is even in unlikely foods, such as savoury dishes and sauces. It is almost true to say that the more sugar there is in a food the better it sells.

It is also true to say that the more sugar you eat the more problems you are creating for yourself in many different parts of your body including your bones. Sugar can lead to hypoglycaemia, diabetes, heart problems and many of the degenerative diseases that are so common today. In addition, an increased sugar intake leads to an increased loss of calcium in urine, leading directly to the problems of osteoporosis.

You do not need sugar, no matter how much you crave it. Remember, sugar contains no nutrients. In addition to the health problems to which it contributes there is a further problem. Since you eat a finite number of calories in a day, sugar squeezes other, more nutritious foods out of your diet. Instead of eating fruit or vegetables. you eat sugar and are left nutritionally worse off.

Sugar craving

Some people crave sugar and insist they need it, just as drug addicts will tell you they crave and need drugs. This does not justify a claim that drugs are good for you, and it doesn't justify a claim that sugar could be good for you.

As you change your diet and begin to eat more vegetables and more wholegrain foods rather than refined foods and generally increase the nutritional content of your diet, your sugar craving will decrease. You can hasten the process by taking a supplement containing generous amounts of all the B group vitamins, which help to reduce sugar cravings. Look for a B complex that also contains chromium and zinc. These two minerals are important for maintaining normal blood sugar metabolism. If you still crave sugar you can reduce the craving still further by taking a supplement of the amino acid glutamine.

Whole foods

We have talked about grains such as wheat, barley, rye and rice and have suggested that it is extremely unlikely that our cave people ancestors ate them. They are now, however, an entrenched part of the daily diet so let's consider what they have to offer.

The grains do provide a number of important nutrients, vitamins and minerals that your body needs. It is true that these could largely be obtained from vegetables but, provided you eat wholemeal grains and wholemeal grain products, you are getting them from these sources as well. Grains also contain fibre, the indigestible carbohydrate that improves the function of your digestive system and prevents constipation. Again, it is

Sugar in the Cave-age diet?

They did not eat sugar, either, with the exception of small amounts of wild honey, which they may have come across from time to time.

true that vegetables also contain fibre – better fibre than grains – but, again, provided that you eat wholemeal grains and their products they do provide fibre.

Refined foods

Note, however, that the emphasis has been on wholemeal grain products. Eating wholemeal flour does have the above benefits; eating white flour does not. Through processing it has lost the great majority of its content of the various B vitamins. A few are replaced after the refining process, and the law allows these products to be called 'enriched'. However, this is like your bank manager emptying your bank balance, putting back a few pennies and telling you your account has been 'enriched'. You would soon notice the difference. White flour loses above 80 per cent of its trace minerals and virtually all its fibre during the refining process.

White flour, from which a lot of nutrients have been removed, is used in the majority of manufactured foods. These include most cakes, biscuits, buns, cookies, pies and pastries. Similar losses occur when brown rice is converted into white rice.

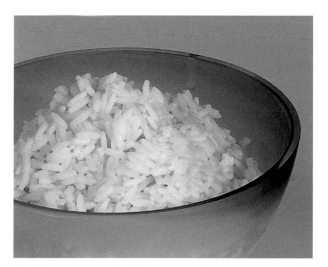

▲ It is recommended that you reduce your intake of refined foods such as white rice and replace them with unrefined versions.

When you eat in restaurants or buy take-away food you will usually find you are eating white (refined) rice, pasta, pastry, breads and other baked goods. Therefore, when you are eating out or buying take-away food, you should try to avoid foods that contain grains or flour. At home you have choice. You can buy and eat wholemeal rather than refined products, so if you crave pasta, this is the place to eat it. Whenever you can, cut out those refined carbohydrates, which will harm your health and weaken your bones, and if you do have to eat refined foods, remember to eat more of a range of vegetables.

Changing your diet

From what we have seen so far, it is clear that the following dietary suggestions should be considered if you want to be healthy and to avoid osteoporosis.

● Consume an adequate but not excessive amount of protein.

● The protein can come from animal sources, such as meat, poultry, fish and eggs, but trim the visible fat from meat; better still eat vegetable proteins.

● Eating a moderate amount of fat is acceptable but it should be unprocessed animal fats or olive oil, not processed margarines, hydrogenated fats or fats that have been cooked or processed to a high temperature.

● Reduce your intake of refined carbohydrates, such as white flour, pasta made with white flour, white rice and sugar.

● Replace the foods you have removed from your diet with greater quantities of fruits and vegetables, particularly vegetables.

Acids and alkalis

Acids and alkalis are opposites, like two sides of a coin, and in general a molecule has an acidic part and an alkaline part. Sometimes the alkaline part is stronger, sometimes the acid part is stronger, resulting in compounds that, overall, are either alkaline or acidic. In addition, when the complex molecules of the foods we eat are broken down, they generally produce a preponderance of alkaline compounds or of acidic compounds.

Foods can be categorized according to whether they leave an acidic or an alkaline residue in the body after they have been eaten. It may seem a little confusing, but this has nothing to do with how acidic or alkaline the foods are before they are consumed. In general, the alkaline-residue foods, those that leave an alkaline ash in the body, have a high content of minerals and are fruits and vegetables. Even seemingly acidic foods, such as tomatoes or oranges, can leave an alkaline residue in the body. The acid-residue foods are meat-based foods and other high-protein foods, fats, grains and sugars. This is true even though they do not seem to be acidic when you eat them.

Acid-residue foods, particularly animal proteins, are known to increase the loss of calcium from the bones and the body in urine, decreasing the amount left behind in bones. This can come about because the acid-forming foods create an acidosis in the blood and, to balance this,

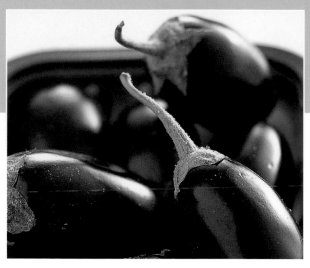

▲ *Make vegetables a significant part of every meal, by serving more unusual vegetables like aubergines with grilled chicken and fish.*

calcium and other minerals may be drawn from bones. Fruit and vegetables have the opposite effect. They can have an alkalizing effect on the blood and do not draw calcium from bones. There are several reasons for this, including the fact that fruits and vegetables have a balanced ratio of calcium to phosphorus, whereas meats, grains and sugars contain more phosphorus than calcium, which can lead to calcium depletion. Another reason is that there is a high level of magnesium in fruits and vegetables.

The ideal diet to prevent or reduce the development of osteoporosis is one that is high in alkaline-residue foods, such as fruits and vegetables, and low in acid-residue foods, such as sugars, grains and refined carbohydrates, and that contains a moderate amount of animal protein.

Vegetables

Whenever I suggest to someone that they should eat more vegetables, they generally insist that they already eat a lot. When we investigate further it usually transpires that they eat two or three vegetables with their evening meal but have no vegetables for breakfast and very few for lunch, perhaps a bit of lettuce and a slice of tomato in a sandwich. Vegetables almost never feature in any snacks they consume. When I say that someone should eat more vegetables I mean that vegetables and fruit should make up a significant part of every meal and every snack eaten throughout the day.

Acids and alkalis in the Cave-age diet?

The diet of our cave-dwelling ancestors was almost certainly a great deal richer in alkaline-residue fruit and vegetable foods and contained far fewer acid-residue foods than does the modern diet.

Vegetables in the Cave-age diet?

It is almost certain that our ancestors ate large amounts of leafy foods. They are easy to collect and easy to eat.

The next question I am usually asked is: 'Which vegetables are the best?' It is tempting to say that it doesn't matter: any vegetable is so much better for you than cakes, biscuits, chocolates, sweets, toffees, crisps (which are often more than 50 per cent fat), mayonnaise or cream and all the other acid-residue foods you are currently eating that you should allow yourself a free choice. However, some vegetables do contain more nutrients and more of the minerals your bones need than others (see tables on pages 122–25).

In the meantime, and before we discuss different vegetables, we need to learn more about the relative roles played by the main minerals in your bones. We need to learn more about calcium, magnesium and phosphorus and the amounts of them that occur in various foods.

Assessing the nutrient content of foods

In any one day the amount of food you eat determines your total calorie intake, which is made up from the calories contained in a combination of foods. In general, if you need, say, 2,000 calories a day to maintain your normal body weight, that is approximately what you will eat every day. If you eat less you will feel hungry; if you eat more you will feel that you have eaten too much. You do not eat a specific weight of food a day – you do not, for instance, say that you must eat a kilogram (about 2lb) of food a day. As soon as you think about it in these terms, it is obvious that this would be wholly impracticable: 1kg (2lb) of cheese, for instance, would be a lot more filling than 1kg (2lb) of lettuce or apples, and your body – and your appetite – would soon tell you so.

When you are assessing the nutrient content of a food and are thinking about nutrient-dense or nutrient-rich foods, it is more important to look for foods that have a high content of the nutrient per calorie that the food provides than its nutrient per 100g (3½oz) of the food. Unfortunately, nearly all nutritional information is given on a per weight basis.

For our purposes we need to know the amount of calcium, magnesium and phosphorus in a fixed number of calories of the various foods. You will find this information in the tables on pages 122–25 .

Sources of calcium

If we consider the amount of calcium in a range of different foods you may be in for some surprises. Many vegetables actually contain more calcium than milk or other dairy products do.

Table 1 shows that on the usual per weight basis various dairy products fall within the top-21 foods and that Cheddar and Camembert cheeses are at numbers one and two. This would suggest that dairy products in general are, indeed, a rich source of calcium. Nuts would also seem to be a rich source, with three of them in the top nine of the foods listed. But consider how many calories you would have to consume to get this calcium; you would have to eat 632 calories of hazelnuts to get 188mg of calcium but only 21 calories of watercress to get slightly more, 192mg.

Table 2 may surprise you. When measured on a per calorie basis – that is, listing the foods by the ones that give you the most calcium for an intake of 100 calories – the cheeses have fallen to numbers 16 and 27 respectively. Cottage cheese has dropped from 21 to 40. Almonds have dropped from 5 to 46, hazelnuts from 8 to 53 and Brazil nuts from 9 to 56. Even buckwheat, which many people consider to be a grain (although it actually belongs in the rhubarb family) has sunk from 16 to 51.

You will see that many vegetables, mostly those with dark green leaves, contain considerably more calcium than milk, some of them more than twice as much. No wonder you were told as a child to eat your greens. Many other vegetables contain nearly as much calcium as milk. Overall, notice that, other than the dairy products (considerably reduced in value), all the foods in the top-31 are vegetables and all those in the top-44 are fruits or vegetables. The nuts, dried beans, meats, grains, fats and sugar that make up the bulk of most people's diets are at the bottom of the calcium supply list.

The benefits of vegetables

Vegetables are an excellent source of calcium and are known to be alkalising your diet. However, they also offer much more. They are an excellent source of many different vitamins, especially of the carotenes that are converted into vitamin A, and of vitamin C and associated bioflavonoids; they also contain many of the B vitamins. Vegetables are an excellent source of minerals, including calcium, magnesium and many of the trace elements needed by your whole body in general and by your bones in particular.

Even the vegetables that do not contain as much calcium as the dairy products contain a lot more than is found in most meats, fish, poultry, grains, nuts, beans, sugar and other commonly eaten foods. This is important to keep in mind as we discuss the other minerals below.

Sources of magnesium

Recall from earlier that your diet should contain nearly as much magnesium as calcium. From Table 3 (see pages 122–23) you will see that nuts and grains are fairly near the top. But, again, you have to consider just how many calories you would be consuming. Table 4 (see pages 122–23) shows that, apart from sunflower seeds, the top 29 foods on a per calorie basis are vegetables. Notice also that to find dairy products, the foods often focused on by those hoping to prevent osteoporosis, you have to go down to the bottom third of the list. You will also see that significant amounts of magnesium are found in a wide range of foods.

Minerals in the 'cave-age' diet?

In cave age times the usual amount of the high-phosphorus foods in the diet was relatively small, consisting mainly of the flesh foods our forebears were able to kill or scavenged. Most of the rest of their diet, largely vegetables and fruits, contained foods with a more equal balance and a preponderance of calcium. The absolute amount of the minerals in flesh foods is small, relative to the amounts in the vegetables. This means that overall there was a high chance that the overall diet worked out to somewhere close to an equal intake of the two.

Table 6 (see pages 124–25) shows the ratio of magnesium to calcium in a range of foods. Ideally, this ratio should be at least 0.5:1, possibly higher. Where are the dairy products? Right at the bottom of the list. Dairy products do provide you calcium but only a negligible amount of magnesium, thus significantly upsetting the important balance of these two minerals.

It is worth reiterating that magnesium is very important for your bones and that it is all too often ignored, holding back the progress some people are expecting when they simply take a calcium supplement and are told, by their doctor or by friends and family, to eat dairy products.

Sources of phosphorus

We have discussed the importance of having a diet that provides approximately equal amounts of phosphorus and calcium (see page 37). Certainly your phosphorus intake should not greatly exceed your calcium intake, or increased amounts of calcium can be lost in urine.

It is worth looking at the phosphorus content of foods, particular at their calcium–to–phosphorus ratio. This time we will skip the list of foods that contain large amounts of phosphorus and move straight to the comparison of the phosphorus–to–calcium ratio

You will see from Table 7 (see pages 124–25) that the foods in the bottom third of the list – that is, those with

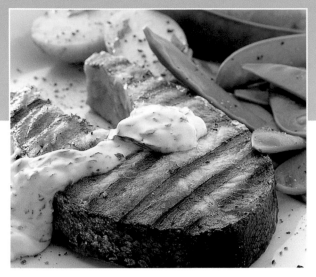

▲ *Salmon has one of the highest ratios of phosphorus to calcium, which can be greatly improved by eating the bones in tinned salmon.*

a relatively low amount of calcium in proportion to the amount of phosphorus they contain – are mainly meats, grains, nuts and seeds. Most of these are 'good' foods, although we have already discussed the role of grains. They contain valuable protein that you need, but your diet almost certainly contains an excessive amount of these foods and an excessive amount of phosphorus compared to calcium. To treat or prevent osteoporosis it is now time to redress this balance.

The top half of Table 7 – that is, the foods that give you the most calcium in proportion to phosphorus – consists entirely of vegetables, fruits and dairy products.

Ratios can be confusing to interpret. In particular, when you go below a 1:1 ratio, the differences between the different fractions seem to be tiny. Yet their significance is large. To demonstrate this, to clarify a few points and to note some interesting figures, look at Table 8 (see pages 124–25). You will see that the highest ratios of phosphorus to calcium are found in flesh foods and that the highest ratio, 23.25:1, is found in salmon. This figure can be improved on if, when you eat tinned salmon, you eat the bones, too. Most of the high-protein meat, poultry and fish foods contain ratios of 15.1:1 or above. Nuts and seeds generally contain at least three times as much phosphorus as calcium and up to 12 times as much. Now you can see that the imbalance in favour of phosphorus is strong. This further emphasizes the need

Minerals in your diet

What does our understanding of the importance of calcium, phosphate and magnesium on bones mean in practice? It means that many of the foods you are probably currently eating contain too much phosphorus, too little calcium and too little magnesium. If grains, cereals, bread, cakes, biscuits, animal proteins and, possibly, nuts or seeds make up the majority of your diet you could be in trouble in at least three ways:

● you are probably on a low-calcium diet
● it is almost certain that you are taking in too much phosphorus and increasing the amount of calcium that is lost from your body and your bones, thereby making the situation worse
● you may or may not be getting the correct ratio of magnesium to calcium, depending on your individual food choices

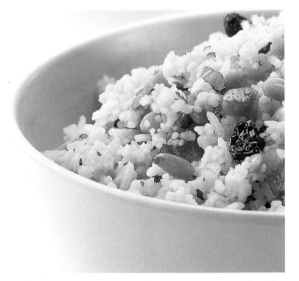

▲ *If your diet consists of a large amount of grains you could be in danger of having a low-calcium diet, having too much phosphorus and not getting the correct ratio of magnesium to calcium.*

for you to eat only moderate amounts of the dense, acid-forming foods, the high-protein flesh foods, high-starch grains and generous amounts of fruits and vegetables.

Sources of trace minerals

Vegetables are also an excellent source of the other trace minerals your bones need. On a per-calorie basis, vegetables in general come out at or near the top of the list of trace mineral-rich foods. It was not the intention of the above section to focus your attention on vegetable foods. It was the discussion of the mineral ratios in foods that kept pointing us to vegetables as being of major benefit in the diet.

Vegetables, it turns out, are the foods that can offer you the best protection from osteoporosis. With this in mind we will look specifically at the different types of vegetable. Think of their mineral content, the beneficial amounts of calcium and magnesium and the moderate amounts of phosphorus, and eat your vegetables, lots of them, increasing the total quantity you consume at every meal. Scrambled egg or an omelette for breakfast could include a variety of vegetables and be served on a bed of mashed

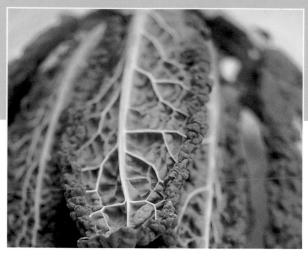

▲ *To ensure that you have several different vegetables for your evening meal, try a selection of carrot mash, cabbage and broccoli to accompany fish or meat.*

carrot or parsnip. For lunch have a salad that contains a wide range of raw vegetables, chopped or grated, not just the usual lettuce and tomatoes and a couple of slices of cucumber. Serve several different vegetables for dinner and have a small salad on the side. If you eat in restaurants, have a salad or plate of vegetables for your first course instead of a calorie-laden, mineral-poor prawn cocktail or some other protein in a creamy sauce. Snack on carrot or celery sticks. It's not only your bones that will benefit: your total health will also improve.

If eating vegetables for breakfast is too radical a change, at least make fruit the major component, with a small amount of more sustaining food, such as a grain or some dairy product. You will find recipes later on in the book. Look particularly at the recipe for Original Fresh Fruit Muesli (see page 66).

Vegetables to avoid

Most people with arthritis already know that vegetables in the Solanaceae (nightshade) family, which includes potatoes, tomatoes, peppers (chillies, paprika and sweet peppers of various colours) and aubergines (eggplants) are not good for them and that they can, over time, aggravate their problem. Some people even feel a distinct worsening of their arthritic symptoms almost immediately they have eaten a large amount of them. Many people have experienced the converse effect: by avoiding these vegetables for a while they gradually find their arthritis is less troublesome.

Vegetable carbohydrates

The macro components of all foods are proteins, fats and carbohydrates. Vegetables contain very little fat, very small amounts of protein and relatively large amounts of carbohydrates. There are three main types of carbohydrates in vegetables:
o starch
o various non-digestible carbohydrates, colloquially called fibre, which are very good for the digestive system
o small amounts of sugar, particularly in fruits such as tomatoes and sweet red peppers

It has also been suggested that these foods and the alkaloid compounds they contain may specifically interfere with calcium metabolism. They may cause calcium to leach from bones, thus causing many of the symptoms of arthritis. For the same reason they may also contribute to the development of osteoporosis.

There is another point that may also be a contributory factor for osteoporosis. As a group, these vegetables have a relatively high phosphorus content and a relatively low calcium content. This is particularly true for potatoes. The ratio of phosphorus to calcium for potato is 7.57:1, for peppers it is 3:1, for aubergine (eggplant) it is 2.17:1, and for tomatoes it is 2.13:1.

For several reasons, therefore, it would seem wise to limit this group of vegetables in your diet, particularly potatoes. Sweet potatoes (yams) are not in the Solanaceae family, so if you do feel like eating a high-starch vegetable, consider choosing one of the sweet potatoes instead.

Are dairy products important?

Given what we know now, you will probably be wondering if you need milk or dairy products in your diet and, specifically, if you need to consume them to avoid osteoporosis. The answer to both questions is 'no', and this should hardly surprise you after what you have read so far. However, there is still more to say about dairy products.

No animal consumes milk or dairy products once the young of the species is weaned. They may do so if it is given to them by a human being, as happens to many pets, but in their natural state none of them do, and osteoporosis is not a serious complaint among wild animals. Animals that are herbivores get sufficient amounts of calcium and other minerals from the grass and other green foods they consume, and we could do the same from vegetables. Carnivorous animals get their calcium, magnesium and other minerals from the bones they chew. Omnivorous animals get theirs from a combination of the sources. As humans, however, we miss out both ways. We do not chew bones with sufficient energy to extract a significant amount of calcium, and we do not eat sufficient quantities of vegetables.

The consumption of dairy products can lead to other problems. First, many people have unsuspected or masked food allergies or sensitivities. These allergies can cause a wide range of generalized symptoms, but they do so over a period of time, so there is no obvious connection between eating the food and developing the symptoms, which are usually prolonged and chronic. The only way you can know about them is to have a specific test done. Dairy products are high among the top ten list of allergenic foods, so if you do have masked food sensitivities there is a good chance that dairy foods are on your list.

Second, people with thrush or who are suffering from candidiasis will benefit from cutting lactose, the milk sugar, out of their diet. Conversely, if they consume milk their thrush can get worse.

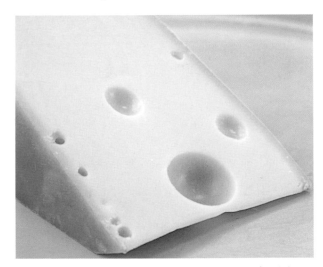

▲ *While dairy products are a good source of calcium, vegetables may be better and offer more protection against osteoporosis.*

Third, many people, even if they are not specifically allergic to dairy products, find that they cause a build-up of unwanted mucus. It may be mild, leading only to some catarrh in the throat that needs the occasional cough or throat-clearing to remove it. Or it may be severe and lead to glue ear in children, infected sinusitis and blinding headaches, poor hearing or a tendency to snore.

For all these reasons, dairy products have little to add to a good diet. For many people not only is milk not the preferred source of calcium, but it could actually be contributing to other health problems. If you are one of the lucky people – and you don't have candidiasis, allergies or suffer from catarrh – judicious amounts of dairy products can be included in your diet, and you will find them in several of the recipes in Part 3 (see pages 64–91).

Few people actually eat a good diet, and few people eat enough vegetables. If you were to double, triple or even quadruple your intake of vegetables you might still not

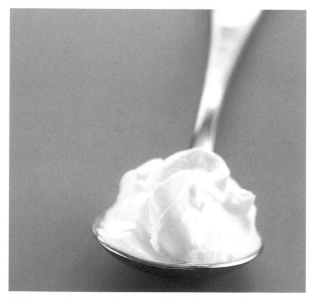

▲ *Natural yogurt is an excellent dairy product to add to your everyday diet, but you should also eat more calcium-rich vegetables.*

be eating enough, and few people are willing to make such a radical dietary change, no matter how good it would be for their bones. If milk is not a problem for you, a compromise plan would seem to be to increase your intake of vegetables as much as you are willing and add some dairy products, particularly natural yogurt, to increase your calcium intake. If you do this, however, you will almost certainly benefit from taking a mineral supplement that gives you generous amounts of magnesium and the other trace minerals to go with the calcium.

Isoflavones

Soya beans contain a range of compounds called isoflavones, which have been found to increase bone density and to be beneficial in preventing osteoporosis. As a fortunate side effect, particularly since most people concerned about osteoporosis are women going through the menopause, they can also help to reduce the hot flushes and some of the other symptoms that occur at this time in a woman's life.

If you do not eat soya beans or soy products you can buy nutritional supplements containing isoflavones. A daily intake of 90–100 mg has been found to be required to make a significant difference to bone density.

Soya beans

Soya beans can be eaten boiled, with or without sauces. They can be sprouted or the flour can be used in a variety of dishes. You can buy soy products such as tofu and tempeh made from fermented soya beans, either plain, smoked, or variously flavoured with different herbs or soy sauce, or a variety of products such as burgers, sausages and other savoury dishes made from cooked soya beans.

Ipriflavone

Ipriflavone is synthesized from one of the soya bean isoflavones. It has been tested in many clinical trials and used extensively in the treatment of osteoporosis. All the evidence is positive. It helps to prevent and treat osteoporosis and does so without any of the adverse side effects of many medical drugs or treatments.

The effect of ipriflavone is two-fold. It is known to reduce bone breakdown and increase bone-building (drugs usually do one or the other which is less effective). Animal tests have shown that it can increase the bones resistance to breaking by as much as 50 per cent. The result is even better when vitamin K is combined with the ipriflavone.

Ipriflavone has many benefits similar to those provided by oestrogen, without any of its harmful side effects. One of the concerns about oestrogen medication is that it can combine with the oestrogen receptor sites in the breasts and thus increase the risk of the person developing breast cancer. There is no evidence that ipriflavone does this, although it does increase the beneficial effect of the oestrogen that you do produce, even after the menopause. This also means that if you do want to take oestrogen, as HRT, then you can make it more effective and use less of it if you take ipriflavone at the same time. Ipriflavone is particularly useful for treating post-menopausal women who may not respond to nutrient supplementation on its own. Some medical treatments induce a temporary condition similar to that of the menopause. All the symptoms of the menopause can occur, as well as decreasing bone density. Taking ipriflavone at the same time has been found to inhibit these effects. Such situations include: the treatment of endometriosis and uterine fibroids and a hysterectomy involving the loss of the ovaries.

Ipriflavone has been used successfully in the treatment of osteoporosis caused by a variety of problems other than increasing age such as long-term periods of immobilization following an accident. Ipriflavone has been shown to decrease this bone loss and sometimes increase bone density even while the bones are inactive.

The long-term use of certain steroid drugs can lead to osteoporosis and diminished bone density. If ipriflavone is taken at the same time it has been shown that this bone loss can be prevented and bone density can actually increase. It has been helpful in the treatment of other diseases in which osteoporosis is a possible consequence. This list includes hyperparathyroidism, Paget's disease, some cases of low-tone tinnitus resulting from otosclerosis and kidney failure involving abnormalities in the metabolism of calcium, phosphorus, vitamin D and parathyroid hormone.

Clearly ipriflavone has many benefits to offer. Remember that it is synthesized from the natural isoflavones that occur in soya beans. These have beneficial effects and so eating soy foods is helpful, but it will not give you ipriflavone which, however, can be obtained as a nutritional supplement from health food shops.

Ipriflavone supplementation is usually in the range of 400–600 mg per day. Take it with meals as this increases the amount you absorb.

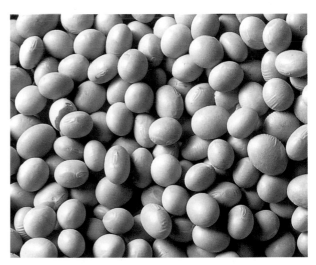

▲ *Soya beans have many positive qualities that improve overall health, not least that they can provide generous amounts of isoflavones and ipriflavones that are known to increase bone density.*

What You Need To Do

Beneficial habits

- Buy organically grown and prepared foods wherever possible; if you can't get organic products do what you can to minimize your consumption of added chemicals.
- Base your diet around vegetables and fruit, especially vegetables, preferably organically grown.
- Use a mineral-rich broth for soups (see page 71).
- Eat a moderate amount of animal protein, including eggs, combined with soya beans, soya products, such as tofu and tempeh, and other plant proteins.
- Where appropriate cook meat on the bone and nibble the flesh off them to extract some of the calcium. If you are eating tinned fish be sure to eat the bones as well (they are usually very soft).
- Maintain a reasonable fat intake, mainly from flesh foods (without the visible fats) and plant sources, such as olives, raw nuts and avocados.
- Use olive oil for cooking and salad dressings.
- Reduce your intake of grains in all forms.
- Give up refined (white) grains in favour of their wholemeal counterparts.
- Give up sugar and sugar-laden foods.
- Reduce your intake of dairy products and, when you have them, focus on natural yogurt and choose full-cream rather than skimmed-milk products.
- Cut out tea, coffee, chocolate and cola.
- Eat less salt.
- Drink only moderate amounts of alcohol – no more than one or two glasses a day.
- Drink eight or more glasses of water a day. If fruits, vegetables and soups make up most of your diet this amount could be reduced slightly as these foods contain considerable amounts of water.
- Avoid soft and carbonated drinks, which may contain caffeine, phosphorus or both.
- Wherever possible avoid medical drugs, particularly the corticosteroids.
- Include weight-bearing exercises and activities in your normal daily routine as well as by participating in planned exercise sessions (see pages 92–121).

Healthy rewards

The changes suggested here may not produce a diet exactly like that of our Cave-age ancestors, with 80 per cent of vegetables and fruits together with some low-fat, lean flesh foods with nuts, herbs and possibly some olive oil. Some of my patients have stuck to such a diet and felt wonderful as a result, but not many are willing to go the full way as it is seen as quite an upheaval. The dietary recommendations outlined here constitute a compromise, but they are probably as far as you are willing to go. It is almost certainly a better diet than you are eating now and will certainly be of great benefit to your bones.

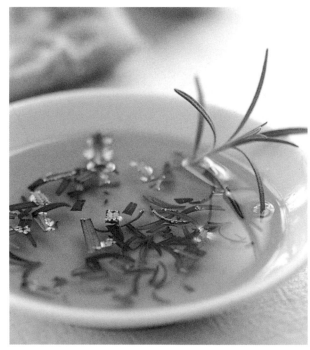

▲ *Olive oil contains essential fatty acids that are beneficial to the diet and should be used in place of other oils in dressings and in cooking generally.*

Your nutritional needs

In an ideal world you would get all the nutrients you need from your diet, but it is unlikely that you will because:

° you probably won't eat the Cave-age diet consisting of two-thirds or more of fruits and vegetables and one-third or less of lean, low-fat protein

° you will be eating food that has been grown and harvested from soils that may be lacking in many of the different minerals your body and bones need, which means that the foods, too, will have less than optimum amounts of these minerals

° your food will have been harvested before it is fully ripe, to allow time for it to be taken to the market and sold before it goes bad; as a result, the full production of vitamins by the plant has not been reached

° your food has almost certainly been picked some considerable time before you eat it, during which time significant amounts of many of the vitamins will have broken down

° the food you eat will have often been prepared in ways in which many of the minerals are lost – for instance, in the cooking water

° many of your lifestyle habits will increase your needs for essential nutrients over and above the needs of our Cave-age ancestors

° pollution and other toxins increase your need for protective nutrients

Do the best you can with your diet. Consider taking supplements to top up your intake as needed, making sure that the supplements provide the various nutrients discussed above and in the appropriate proportions.

These suggestions may seem to be pretty radical. When you look at this list you may think you have so many changes to make that the process is impossible. If that is the case and if you are suffering from osteoporosis, you may have identified a major part of the cause. It could be your diet that has caused much of the problem.

Keep in mind that osteoporosis is much more common in the Western world than in developing countries, where diets do not include all our modern, Western, processed foods. People in developing countries generally eat fewer sugars and soft drinks, less refined white flour, fewer high saturated-fat products such as roast (in oil) nuts and crisps. In fact, they generally adhere more closely to the above indications than people in the West do.

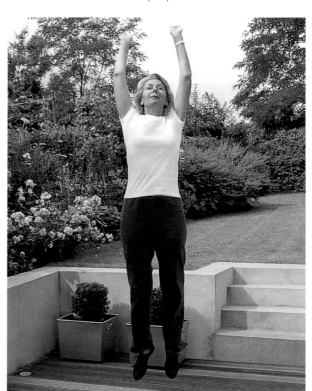

▲ *An extra benefit of changing your diet to ensure you are receiving maximum levels of the right nutrients and vitamins is that you will also increase your energy.*

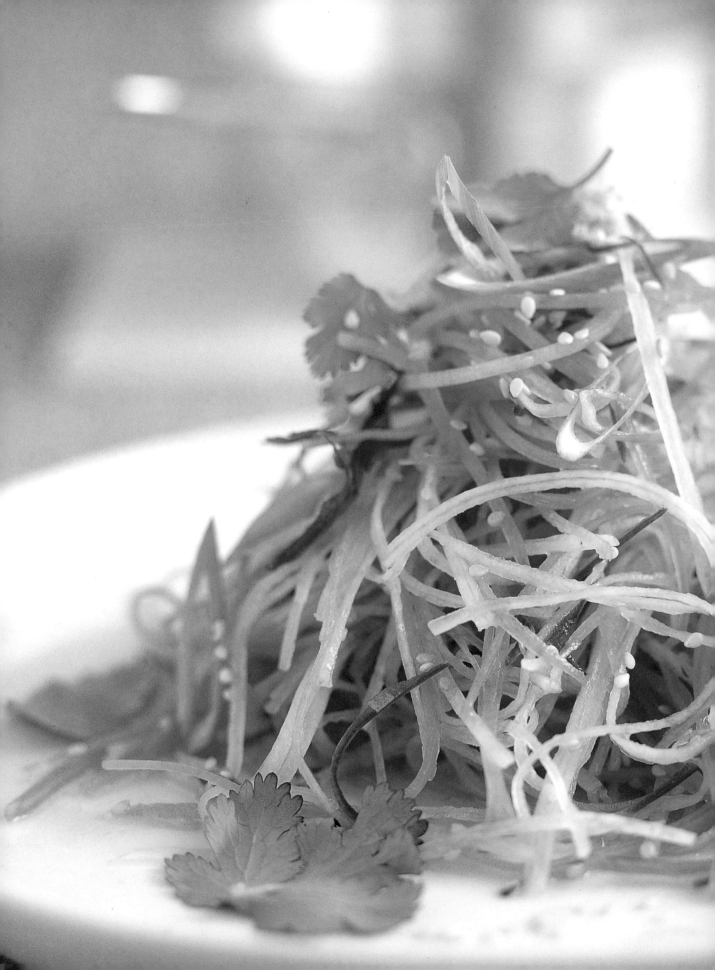

Recipes

3

This is not intended to be a comprehensive recipe book. Instead, the emphasis has been placed on dishes that are relatively rich in the nutrients needed by your bones, particularly vegetable dishes. You may be surprised to find that they can be a lot more fun that you had thought. Even meat-based dishes can include a wide range of mineral-rich vegetables.

I suggest you base your meals on fresh vegetables and use meat and whatever starch food you choose, such as pasta or rice, as accompaniments. Use the recipes and suggestions given here to stimulate your own thinking – and remember the Cave-age diet.

Original Fresh Fruit Muesli

This is an excellent meal with which to start the day. You will get carotenes (for vitamin A) from the fruits, B vitamins from the oats, yogurt and sunflower seeds, vitamin C from the fruits and vitamin E from the seeds. You will get minerals from the yogurt, oats and seeds and fibre from the fruit, oats and seeds. Finally, you will get essential fatty acids from the seeds and protein from the yogurt, oats and seeds. Best of all, perhaps, you will get short-term energy from the sugars in the fruits, long-term energy from the starches in the oats and even longer-term energy from the fats in the seeds. As a result, this original muesli will see you safely through a busy morning and satisfy you until lunchtime. If by any chance it doesn't, then simply eat more of it, do not change the proportions.

Serves: 2
Preparation time: 10 minutes

2 tablespoons raw porridge oats
2 tablespoons full-fat milk
½ cup strawberries
½ cup raspberries
1 apple, chopped
1 banana, chopped
200ml (7fl oz) full-fat natural yogurt
1 tablespoon raw almonds, chopped
1 tablespoon sunflower seeds

1 Place the oats in a bowl and moisten with the milk. You can allow this to soak if you wish or prepare it immediately prior to serving. Add the fresh fruits. Pour over the natural yogurt. Sprinkle the chopped nuts and seeds on top.

Smoothies

Smoothies, consisting simply of fruits, will provide vitamin C and the bioflavonoids and pycnogenols, all good antioxidants. You can make a variety of fruit smoothies. Simply combine your chosen fruits in a blender and blend until smooth. Add ice cubes if you like a cool drink and decorate with mint leaves. Add milk or yogurt if you like creamy drinks, but remember to make it full-fat milk or yogurt so you can efficiently absorb the calcium that it contains.

If you want something to get your teeth into, add nuts or seeds. For example, put some almonds into the blender, then the fruit, and blend until smooth. This will add some minerals and essential fatty acids. It will also, of course, increase the calorie content significantly.

Smoothies are particularly useful if you are in a hurry in the morning. However, you should remember that they are foods, rather than drinks, and you should sip them slowly, allowing them to mix with plenty of saliva before swallowing, and you should chew them well if you have added nuts or seeds.

Eggs Florentine

*Spinach leaves are a good source of iron and other minerals and combine with the calcium in
the cheese. Spinach is also a source of carotenes, B vitamins, vitamin C and the associated
antioxidant bioflavonoids and pycnogenols and vitamin K. Eggs are a low-calorie source of
protein with the highest available net utilization. In general, eggs provide more nutrients per
calorie than almost any other food. They are also rich in methionine, an important amino acid
that benefits your liver. Although cream may have more appeal, a thick Greek-style yogurt
would provide better nutrition.*

Serves: 4
Preparation time: 3 minutes
Cooking time: 15 minutes

500g (1lb) spinach leaves, without stems
2 tablespoons thin cream
4 eggs
4 slices Swiss cheese
salt and freshly ground black pepper to taste

1 Wash the spinach leaves, shake lightly and place in a
dry saucepan. Put the lid on and cook over gentle
heat. When cooked, squeeze, drain off the excess
liquid and chop the leaves finely. Add the cream,
season and place in an ovenproof dish.

2 Poach the eggs in gently simmering water. When
cooked, place them on the bed of spinach. Cover
each one with a slice of Swiss cheese and place the
dish in a hot oven or under a warm grill until the
cheese has melted.

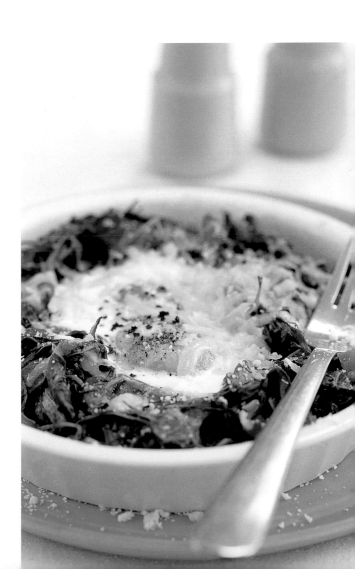

Watercress Soup

Watercress leaves are a good source of iron and other minerals and combine with the calcium in the cheese. The milk and yogurt add calcium and protein and the yogurt improves your digestive system by adding the beneficial flora.

Serves: 4
Preparation time: 5 minutes
Cooking time: 20 minutes

250g (8oz) potatoes
600ml (1 pint) water or vegetable stock
2 generous bunches watercress, finely chopped
milk, to the desired texture
natural yogurt to decorate
salt and pepper

1 Cook the potatoes in the water or stock until tender; cool and blend. Reheat the puréed potato, add the watercress and simmer gently for 5 minutes.

2 Add sufficient milk to give you the degree of thickness you require. Season to taste and serve with a swirl of natural yogurt.

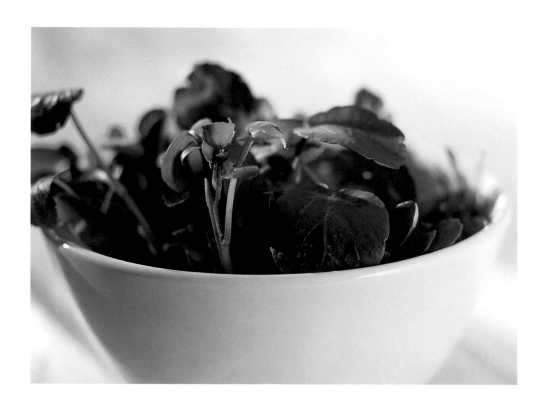

Broccoli and Cheese Soup

The minerals in the broccoli combine well with the calcium in the cheese and yogurt. Broccoli is a good source of vitamin K, carotenes and other antioxidant nutrients such as vitamin C, the bioflavonoids and pycnogenols. It is a good source of fibre if you include generous amounts of the stems, and the yogurt will help your digestive system.

Serves: 6
Preparation time: 10 minutes
Cooking time: 20 minutes

1kg (2lb) broccoli
50g (2oz) butter or olive oil
1 onion, chopped
1 large potato, peeled and quartered
1.5 litres (2½ pints) vegetable stock
1 tablespoon lemon juice
1 teaspoon Worcestershire sauce
few drops Tabasco sauce, or to taste
125ml (4fl oz) natural yogurt
125g (4oz) mature Cheddar cheese, grated
salt and pepper
sprigs of watercress, to garnish

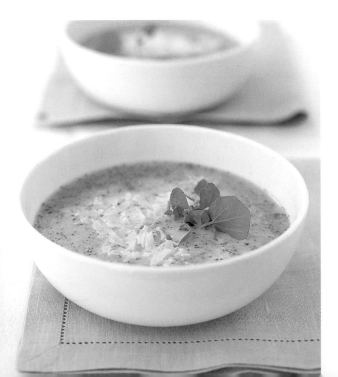

1 Remove all the very tough stems and leaves from the broccoli. (These can be used in making basic stock; see page 71.) Cut off the stalks, peel them and cut, crossways, into thin slices. Break the florets into small pieces and set them aside.

2 Melt the butter in a large saucepan. Add the onion and broccoli stalks and cook, covered, for 5 minutes over a moderate heat. Stir frequently.

3 Add the broccoli florets, potato and vegetable stock to the pan. Bring the mixture to the boil and cook, partially covered, for 5 minutes. Use a slotted spoon to remove 6 or more florets for a garnish and set aside. Season the mixture with salt and pepper and continue to cook over a moderate heat for a few minutes until all the vegetables are just soft.

4 Use a blender or food processor and purée the mixture in batches until smooth, transferring each successive batch to a clean saucepan. Add the lemon juice, Worcestershire sauce and a few drops of Tabasco sauce to the pan. Simmer for 3–5 minutes. Stir in the yogurt.

5 Just before serving, stir in the grated cheese and garnish each portion with the reserved florets and sprigs of watercress.

Sweet Potato, Leek and Coriander Soup

Earlier we discussed the benefits of sweet potato over potato tubers. Because this recipe replaces potatoes with sweet potatoes, it is an excellent choice for people with arthritis or other joint problems that might be aggravated by vegetables from the nightshade family. Sweet potatoes also contain more carotenes than the more common potatoes. The yogurt adds calcium and protein and helps your digestive system and leeks are a good source of calcium and magnesium.

Serves: 4
Preparation time: 10 minutes
Cooking time: 25 minutes

1 tablespoon olive oil
1 teaspoon black mustard seeds
1 onion, finely chopped
1 garlic clove, crushed
500g (1lb) sweet potatoes, diced
1 litre (1¾ pints) mineral-rich stock (some of this can be replaced by milk if preferred, in which case it should be added at the end)
3 small leeks, trimmed, cleaned and finely sliced
sprigs of fresh coriander, to taste
salt and pepper
natural yogurt, to garnish

1 Warm the olive oil in a heavy-based saucepan. Add the mustard seeds, onion, garlic and sweet potatoes. Cook for 5 minutes. Add the stock, bring to the boil and simmer gently for about 10 minutes or until the sweet potato is tender.

2 Add the leeks. Chop and add the coriander. Simmer for another 5 minutes. Season to taste. Serve with a swirl of natural yogurt in the centre.If you prefer, blend the soup before serving.

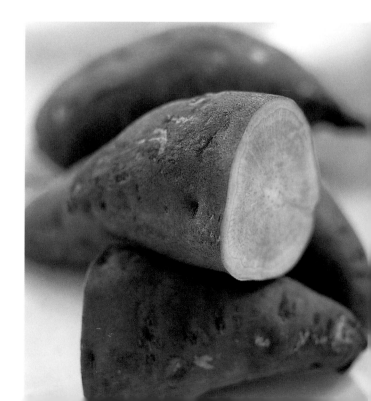

Stocks

Meat Stock

Bones make an excellent basis for a soup stock, and can be cooked for as long as you like. Ideally they should be from organically reared or wild animals. In addition to the flavours they provide they are a source of calcium and other minerals. These are leached out more readily if some acid is added to the stock liquid, hence the use of vinegar or wine.

1–1.5kg (2–3lb) bones
3 tablespoons vinegar or oxidized (old) wine

Place the bones in a large saucepan and cover with water. Add the vinegar or wine. Simmer for 3 hours. Instead of animal or chicken bones you can use fishbones or the shells of crustaceans, such as prawns, crabs and lobsters if you have them. You could also add the cleaned and crushed shells of organically produced eggs.

Mineral-rich soup

Soups have their good and bad points. Traditionally the old-fashioned soup pot was placed on the back of the stove, a range of leftovers, cooked and raw, was added over time and it was allowed simmer until it was wanted. This may have resulted, and often did, in a tasty combination, but would have destroyed most of the vitamin content – it would, however, still have been a rich source of minerals (depending on the ingredients used) because heat does not break these down. None the less there are better ways to make nutrient-rich and tasty soups.

Remember to add some vinegar or wine that has turned acidic to the water you use in order to leach out more of the minerals from the bones.

Vegetable Additions

Here is your chance to use the outer unwanted leaves or skin of vegetables. You can use the outer leaves of cabbages, onions, leeks, cauliflower, celery etc, and, if you do peel them, the peelings of carrots, potatoes and other root vegetables. Since you would otherwise be simply throwing these vegetables it is excellent that you will now be boiling them for a long time, extracting as much of the mineral content as possible. You will destroy the vitamins in the process so be sure to add plenty of fresh fruit, salads and lightly cooked vegetables to your diet to ensure an adequate intake of these.

Add these vegetable ingredients, finely chopped, to the strained meat stock liquid and simmer the mixture for the last half hour. If you are a vegetarian you will start simply with the vegetable ingredients, using no bones.

Whichever stock you have made, once it is cooked, strain, pressing all the water out of the cooked vegetables, and allow it to cool. Chill in the fridge and, if using bones or meat offcuts, skim off any fat that comes to the top. Use the stock as the basis for quick-cook soups. The liquid can be frozen and used at a later date.

Sweet Potato and Grilled Chilli Salad

Sweet potatoes make an interesting alternative to usual potato tubers. People with arthritis or related problems, who want to avoid ordinary potatoes, will find them just as versatile as the more common varieties. This is a spicy and satisfying salad. Make sure you add all the green leaves to increase the mineral and vitamin content of the dish.

Serves: 4
Preparation time: 20 minutes
Cooking time: 20 minutes

750g (1½lb) sweet potatoes, washed, peeled and sliced
3 large fresh red chillies
6 tablespoons olive oil (for frying)
handful of coriander leaves, torn
coarse sea salt and pepper
100g (3½ oz) lamb's lettuce or rocket

Dressing:
1 teaspoon finely grated lime rind
2 tablespoons lime juice
4 tablespoons olive oil
2 tablespoons sesame oil

1 Parboil the sweet potato slices in a large saucepan of boiling water for 5 minutes. Drain well, then refresh under cold running water. Spread out on kitchen paper to dry.

2 Preheat the grill to hot, and cook the chillies, turning them frequently, until the skins are blistered and blackened all over. Leave to cool slightly, then carefully remove and discard the skin and seeds. Cut the flesh into thin strips and set aside. Wash your hands carefully afterwards to remove any irritant chilli that could sting your eyes or an open cut.

3 Heat 3 tablespoons of olive oil in a large frying pan. Sauté the sweet potato slices in batches over a medium-high heat until crisp and lightly browned. Transfer to a large, shallow serving bowl as they are done and add more oil to the pan as necessary.

4 Make the dressing. Mix all the ingredients together in a small bowl until thoroughly blended, or shake together in a screw-top jar.

5 Add the strips of chilli and the torn coriander leaves to the sweet potatoes in the salad bowl. Season to taste and toss lightly to mix.

6 Just before serving, pour the dressing over the sweet potatoes and chilli and toss well. Serve with lamb's lettuce or rocket.

Vegetable Bites with Dipping Sauce

This dish allows you to use a variety of vitamin- and mineral-rich vegetables. Good ones to choose are peeled broccoli stalks, carrots, cucumber and courgette sticks, French beans, Chinese leaves, cauliflower florets and strips of red, orange and yellow peppers. If you remove the seeds from the chilli pepper wash your hands carefully afterwards. Make sure that you do not rub your eyes before you wash your hands. Tamarind, also known as Indian date, is a sour-tasting fruit, usually sold compressed in blocks. It should be soaked in hot water to extract the flavour. Tamarind can also be bought in paste form, when it should be mixed with sufficient water to give a runny consistency. Lemon juice can be used instead in this recipe, although it has less flavour.

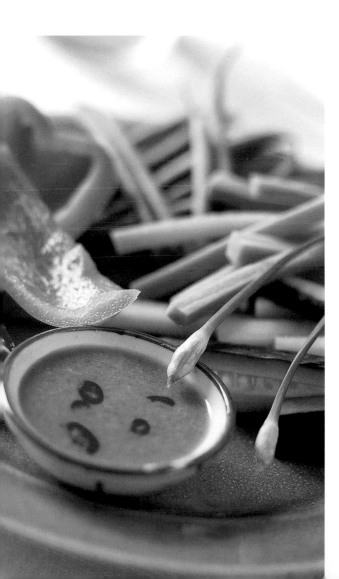

Serves: 4
Preparation time: 15 minutes
Cooking time: 5–6 minutes

about 500g (1lb) vegetables of your choice

Dipping sauce:
125g (4oz) yellow bean sauce
½ onion, chopped
1 tablespoon tamarind (see above)
200ml (7fl oz) coconut milk
200ml (7fl oz) water
2 eggs
2 tablespoons honey
1 tablespoon soy sauce
1 large fresh red chilli, sliced lengthways, to garnish

1 Choose a mixture of raw vegetables and chop them into lengths.

2 To make the dipping sauce: blend the yellow bean sauce and the onion in a blender or food processor and turn into a saucepan. Add the rest of the sauce ingredients and bring gradually to the boil, stirring. Remove from the heat and pour into a bowl.

3 Garnish the prepared sauce with the sliced chilli and serve warm, with the vegetables.

Carrot, Daikon and Red Pepper Salad

Carrots are a source of carotene and high in fibre. Peppers, particularly the red ones, are an excellent source of vitamin C and contain, beneficially, nearly twice as much magnesium as calcium. Sesame seeds contain calcium and several of the B group of vitamins.

Serves: 4
Preparation time: 5–10 minutes
Cooking time: 2–3 minutes

3 carrots
1 small daikon (white radish)
1 large, firm red pepper
1 tablespoon toasted sesame seeds
1 teaspoon sesame oil
1 tablespoon rice wine vinegar
¼ teaspoon coriander powder

To garnish:
4 spring onions, finely shredded
coriander leaves

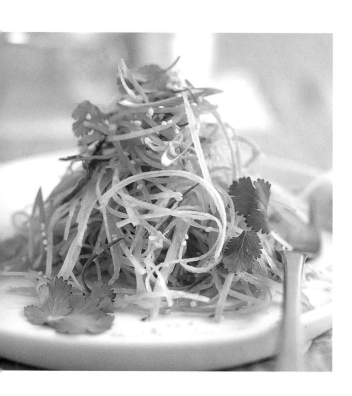

1 Cut the carrots, daikon and red pepper into julienne strips. Alternatively, you can peel them lengthways with a potato peeler. Lightly combine the vegetables and sesame seeds. Divide the mixture into four and arrange on four individual serving plates.

2 Warm the sesame oil, rice wine vinegar and coriander powder to blend the flavours. Allow to cool and pour the dressing over and around the salad. Garnish with spring onions and fresh coriander leaves.

Sweet Potato, Rocket and Haloumi Salad

This is a filling and satisfying salad. It can be served as a light meal in itself or used to accompany other salad dishes with a greater emphasis on raw and leafy, low-calorie vegetables. The calcium in the haloumi cheese combines with the calcium and other minerals in the vegetables to make a nutritious meal. The haloumi provides protein and the sweet potatoes provide bulk and are satisfying. Sweet potatoes are also an excellent choice for people with arthritis or other joint problems that might be aggravated by potatoes of the nightshade family and they contain more carotenes than the more common potatoes. The rocket leaves provide a range of vitamins and minerals including the very important vitamin K.

Serves: 4
Preparation time: 10 minutes
Cooking time: 15 minutes

500g (1lb) sweet potatoes, sliced
3 tablespoons olive oil
250g (8oz) haloumi cheese, patted dry on kitchen paper
100g (3½oz) rocket

Dressing:
5 tablespoons olive oil
3 tablespoons clear honey
2 tablespoons lemon or lime juice
1½ teaspoons black onion seeds
1 red chilli, deseeded and finely sliced
2 teaspoons chopped lemon thyme
freshly ground black pepper

1 Mix together all the ingredients for the dressing in a small bowl. Do not be tempted to add salt because there is plenty in the haloumi cheese.

2 Cook the sweet potatoes in boiling water for 2 minutes and drain well. Heat the oil in a large frying pan, add the sweet potatoes and fry for about 10 minutes, turning once, until golden.

3 Meanwhile, thinly slice the cheese and place on a lightly oiled, foil-lined grill rack. Cook under a preheated moderate grill for about 3 minutes until golden, turning once.

4 Pile the sweet potatoes, cheese and rocket on to serving plates and spoon the dressing over them.

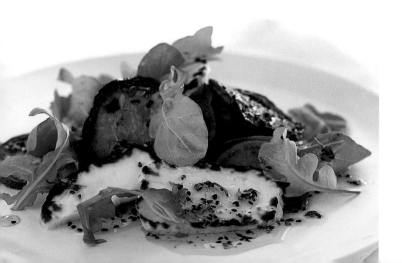

Leftover Salads

Salads are not simply the side dish of leaves served in many restaurants or a combination of lettuce, cucumber, tomato and tinned beetroot. A salad can be any combination of fresh vegetables that you choose, raw, fresh or leftovers. You can have as many salads as your imagination can create.

Adding fruits to a salad can make all the difference between a dull and ordinary salad and one with an unusual and interesting flavour.

A plain-looking salad will become truly eye-catching if you decorate it with fresh herbs or colourful flowers. Nasturtium and borage flowers are not only beautiful but also nutritious. The delicate leaves of fennel and dill or the curls of parsley leaves provide contrasting shapes and textures.

We have already spoken about the high nutrient density of vegetables. This is particularly true of raw vegetables as there is no chance of the vitamins being destroyed during the cooking process or the vitamins or minerals being lost in the cooking water. Put particular emphasis on the dark green, bright red and bright orange vegetables to ensure maximum supply of nutrients such as the B vitamins and the antioxidant vitamins such as the carotenes, vitamin C, bioflavonoids and pycnogenols. Remember the vitamin K to be found particularly in dark green leafy vegetables and broccoli. Add fruits to include vitamin C and more bioflavonoids and pycnogenols.

There is nothing more appealing for a large banquet or buffet than a table spread with a variety of different salads. Vary the textures and colours and you can create an enticing kaleidoscope of dishes. The meat dishes on the side can safely be left to play second fiddle. The dedicated carnivore will certainly find them.

• Start with cold ratatouille, add a small amount of mayonnaise, serve cold on a bed of sliced tomato and you have managed to revitalize an otherwise uninspiring leftover.

• Cold cooked cauliflower or broccoli tossed in a French dressing and decorated with pine nuts is simply delicious.

• Toss cooked carrots in yogurt and decorate with fresh, chopped dill leaves.

• Cooked peas, tossed in an oil and vinegar dressing with chopped mint is refreshing and a good source of protein.

• Treat cooked parsnips or carrots in the same way as you would potato to make a potato salad.

• Other vegetables can be treated in similar ways. Let your imagination run riot.

Preserving nutrients

Do not throw out those vegetable leftovers from a meal. Keep them to eat cold as, or with, salads at the next meal. You can also cook vegetables especially for this dish and allow them to cool. If you do this it is usually better to undercook them slightly so they still retain a certain amount of 'bite'. You can include single vegetables or a dish of cooked mixed vegetables or vegetable stew.

One of the advantages of this method of using up leftover vegetables is that, because you don't have to reheat them, some of the nutrients they contain, especially the vitamins, can be preserved.

Salad Dressings

To focus on your bones and the calcium they need, look out for salad dressings that contain generous amounts of fresh green herbs or that include dairy products such as yogurt or cheese. These are excellent, calcium-rich dressings, which can be added to any salad.

Creamy Blue Cheese Dressing

Using a blue cheese, such as Bleu d'Auvergne, Cashel Blue, Danish Blue or Roquefort, gives the dressing a strong and piquant flavour. Use it with strongly flavoured vegetables to provide contrast or with green salads to add an extra element of taste.

125g (4oz) blue cheese, crumbled
125ml (4fl oz) mayonnaise
125ml (4fl oz) Greek yogurt
large pinch of salt
½ teaspoon pepper

Combine all the ingredients and mix well. Store the dressing in the refrigerator until ready to use.

Lemon and Yogurt Dressing

150g (5oz) natural yogurt
1 tablespoon lemon juice
2 tablespoons chopped mixed fresh herbs
salt and pepper

Combine all the ingredients and mix well. Refrigerate until ready to serve. The acidity of the lemon juice, beneficial organisms in the yogurt and fibre in whatever salad you choose to pour this dressing over will all benefit your digestion.

Variations
Use mint instead of mixed herbs for cucumber or potato salads, basil for tomato salads, dill or fennel leaves on carrot salads and parsley for green salads.

Cottage Cheese Mayonnaise

Cottage cheese is an excellent source of low-calorie protein as well as being a source of calcium. Eggs provide more nutrients per calorie than almost any other food and are also rich in methionine, an important amino acid for your liver.

100g (3½oz) cottage cheese
2 egg yolks
3 tablespoons olive oil
1 teaspoon vinegar or fresh lemon juice
½ teaspoon French or German mustard
fresh herbs and/or seasoning to taste

Place all the ingredients in a blender and blend well. If the mixture is too thick add some natural yogurt to adjust.

Vegetable Rice Pancakes

Who says vegetables are dull? These paper-thin rice pancakes make interesting wraps for a variety of tempting fillings such as this light combination of vegetables. Served with a highly flavoured sauce, they make an intriguing starter to any meal. Allow two rice pancakes for each person; one if there is a heavy meal to follow.

Serves: 4
Preparation time: 15 minutes
Cooking time: 5 minutes

Sauce:
1 garlic clove, roughly chopped
5cm (2in) piece fresh root ginger, peeled and roughly chopped
3 tablespoons light muscovado sugar or honey
4 teaspoons soy sauce
5 teaspoons wine or rice vinegar
2 tablespoons tomato purée
2 tablespoons sesame seeds, plus extra to garnish

Pancakes:
8 rice pancakes
2 medium carrots, cut into fine shreds
100g (3½oz) bean sprouts or mixed sprouting beans
small handful of mint, roughly chopped
1 celery stick, thinly sliced
4 spring onions, thinly sliced diagonally
1 tablespoon soy sauce

1 Place all the ingredients for the sauce, except the sesame seeds, in the small bowl of a food processor or in a blender and process to a thin paste. Alternatively, crush the garlic, grate the ginger and whisk in with the remaining ingredients. Stir in the sesame seeds and transfer to a serving bowl.

2 Soften the rice pancakes; follow the instructions on the packet. Combine the carrots, bean sprouts or sprouting beans, mint, celery, spring onions and soy sauce.

3 Divide the vegetable mixture among the pancakes, spooning it into the middle of each. Fold in the bottom edge of each pancake to the middle, then roll up from one side to the other to form a pocket.

4 Steam the pancakes in a vegetable steamer or bamboo steamer for about 5 minutes until heated through. Alternatively, place on a wire rack set over a roasting tin of boiling water and cover with foil. Serve immediately with the sauce, garnished with sesame seeds.

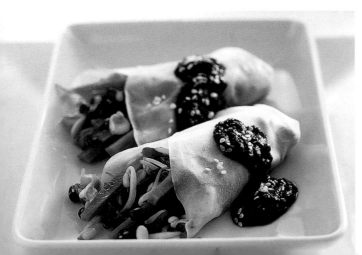

Celeriac and Potato Remoulade

*Make this into a complete meal for a light lunch or supper by lightly poaching some eggs and
arranging them over the asparagus. Celeriac, the root vegetable with a flavour similar to celery,
is a good source of minerals and fibre and the yogurt adds calcium and protein to the dish.*

Serves: 4
Preparation time: 10 minutes
Cooking time: 10 minutes

500g (1lb) celeriac, peeled
375g (12oz) potatoes, peeled
1 tablespoon extra virgin olive oil, plus extra for
drizzling (optional)
500g (1lb) asparagus, trimmed

Sauce:
150ml (¼ pint) mayonnaise
150ml (¼ pint) Greek yogurt
1 teaspoon Dijon mustard
6 cocktail gherkins, finely chopped
2 tablespoons capers, chopped
2 tablespoons chopped tarragon
salt and pepper

1 Cut the celeriac and potatoes into matchstick-sized
pieces. Cook the celeriac in lightly salted boiling
water for 2 minutes or until softened. Add the
potatoes and cook for a further 2 minutes or until
just tender. Drain the vegetables and refresh under
running water.

2 Mix together the ingredients for the sauce and
set aside.

3 Heat the oil in a frying pan or griddle pan. Add the
asparagus and fry for 2–3 minutes until just
beginning to colour. Mix the celeriac and potato
with the sauce and spoon onto 4 serving plates.
Arrange the asparagus spears on top and serve
immediately, drizzled with a little extra olive
oil if wished.

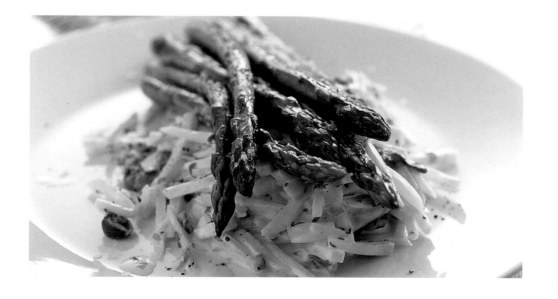

Aubergine Rolls

*The rolls are formed from slices of aubergine cut lengthways. They are filled with a simple,
light mixture of soft goats' cheese and ricotta flavoured with basil, and served on a bed of
diced peppers and rocket with a tomato sauce. This is an excellent protein-rich vegetable dish
that is tasty and satisfying without being too heavy. To make a complete and substantial
meal, serve with steamed brown rice. The peppers and rocket add fibre, vitamins and minerals,
and the ricotta provides calcium.*

Serves: 4
Preparation time: 10 minutes
Cooking time: 25 minutes

4 aubergines, about 250g (8oz) each, thinly
sliced lengthways
olive oil, for brushing
250g (8oz) ricotta cheese
250g (8oz) soft goats' cheese
150g (5oz) Parmesan cheese, freshly grated, plus extra
shavings to serve
4 tablespoons chopped basil
4 large pieces sun-dried tomato in oil, drained and sliced
salt and pepper
diced peppers and rocket to serve
snipped chives or sprigs of basil, to garnish

Tomato sauce:
2 tablespoons olive oil
1 onion, chopped
2 garlic cloves, crushed
1kg (2lb) sun-ripened tomatoes, skinned, deseeded
and chopped
150ml (¼ pint) vegetable or chicken stock, medium dry
white wine or water
about 1 tablespoon sun-dried tomato purée
salt and pepper

1 Make the tomato sauce. Heat the oil in a saucepan,
add the onion and cook gently, stirring
occasionally, until soft. Stir in the garlic, tomatoes,
stock, wine or water, and tomato purée, then
simmer until thickened to a fairly light sauce.
Season to taste.

2 Meanwhile, brush the aubergine slices lightly with
oil. Cook under a preheated grill until evenly
browned on both sides. Drain on kitchen paper.

3 Mix together the ricotta and goats' cheeses,
125g (4oz) of the Parmesan, the chopped basil and
seasoning to taste. Spoon the cheese mixture along
each aubergine slice and add a slice of sun-dried
tomato. Roll the aubergine slices, from the short
end, around the filling. Place the rolls, seam-side
down, in a single layer in a shallow ovenproof dish
and sprinkle with the remaining Parmesan. Place
under a preheated grill for 5 minutes until the
filling is hot.

4 Serve the rolls on a bed of diced peppers and
rocket leaves. Scatter over shavings of Parmesan
and garnish with snipped chives or sprigs of basil.
Reheat the tomato sauce if necessary and serve
separately.

Root Vegetable Bake

These vegetables are a source of many nutrients plus fibre. Watercress, a rich source of minerals and vitamins, and alkalising alfalfa sprouts, would be an alternative garnish. For a creamier texture serve the vegetable bake with a dish of natural yogurt,

Serves: 4
Preparation time: 20 minutes
Cooking time: 40–50 minutes

500g (1lb) new potatoes, washed
250g (8oz) swedes, peeled and cubed
300g (10oz) parsnips, peeled and sliced
250g (8oz) carrots, peeled and cut into sticks
65ml (2½fl oz) vegetable stock (see page 71)
50g (2oz) reduced-fat cheese, preferably Edam or
Cheddar, grated
salt and pepper

To garnish:
tomato slices
1 tablespoon chopped fresh parsley

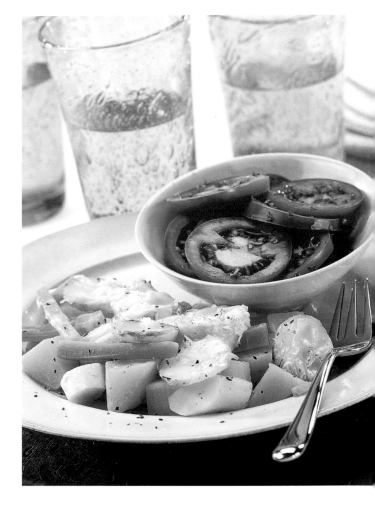

1 Place the potatoes in a pan of boiling water and cook until just tender. Lift out and cut into 5mm (¼in) slices and set aside. Bring the water to the boil again, add the remaining vegetables and simmer until just tender. Drain the vegetables and place in layers in a deep ovenproof dish, alternating with the potatoes and finishing with a border of overlapping potato slices. Pour over the stock, sprinkle with the cheese and season with salt and pepper.

2 Preheat the oven to 180°C (350°F), Gas Mark 4, and bake for 15–20 minutes or until the cheese has melted and the vegetables are heated through. Brown under a moderate grill to finish if wished.

3 Garnish with tomato slices and chopped parsley, if liked.

Stir-fried Vegetables

These stir-fried vegetables may be served as an accompaniment to meat or fish. You can add brown rice if you are hungry, but remember to keep the vegetable component the major part of the meal. These vegetables are at their best when they are lightly cooked and still crunchy. Use fresh bean sprouts as tinned bean sprouts do not have a sufficiently crunchy texture. The vegetables are rich in minerals, vitamins and fibre.

Serves: 4
Preparation time: 15–20 minutes
Cooking time: 3–5 minutes

1 tablespoon olive oil
125g (4oz) bamboo shoots, thinly sliced
50g (2oz) mangetout
125g (4oz) carrots, thinly sliced
50g (2oz) broccoli florets
125g (4oz) fresh bean sprouts, rinsed
1 teaspoon honey
1 tablespoon stock or water
salt and pepper

1 Heat the oil in a preheated wok or frying pan. Add the bamboo shoots, mangetout, carrots and broccoli florets and stir-fry for about 1 minute.

2 Add the bean sprouts with the honey and seasoning. Stir-fry for another minute or so, then add some stock or water if necessary. Do not overcook, or the vegetables will lose their crunchiness. Serve hot.

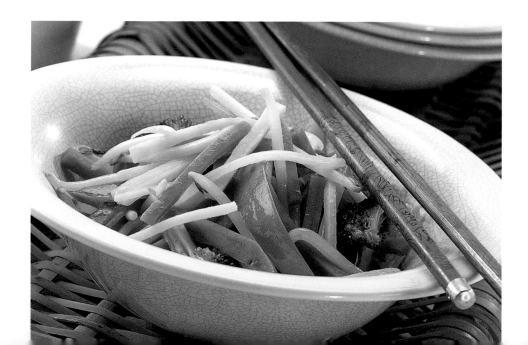

Spicy Roast Vegetables

These lightly spiced roast vegetables are delicious as a starter, a side dish or a finger snack. Although called roast vegetables, they are actually better cooked in a large, heavy-based grill pan. Since the vegetables in this dish are mainly 'fruits', it is not surprising to find it is a source of vitamin C and the associated bioflavonoids and pycnogenols.

Serves: 6
Preparation time: 10 minutes
Cooking time: 15 minutes

2 tablespoons good quality extra virgin olive oil
½ teaspoon white cumin seeds
1 green pepper, cored, deseeded and thickly sliced
1 red pepper, cored, deseeded and thickly sliced
1 orange pepper, cored, deseeded and thickly sliced
2 courgettes, diagonally sliced
2 tomatoes, halved
2 red onions, quartered
1 aubergine, thickly sliced
2 thick fresh green chillies, sliced
4 garlic cloves
2.5cm (1in) piece fresh root ginger, peeled and shredded
1 teaspoon dried, crushed red chillies
½ teaspoon salt

To garnish:
1 tablespoon chopped fresh coriander
lemon wedges

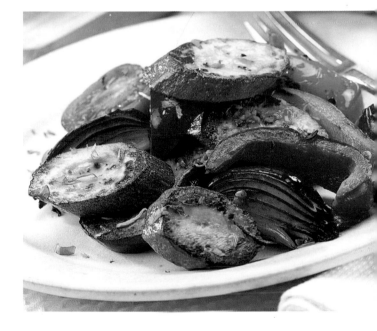

1   Heat the grill pan for 2 minutes. Pour in the olive oil, then add the cumin seeds. Lower the heat to medium.

2   Arrange the vegetables in the pan with a pair of tongs, then add the green chillies, garlic, ginger, red chillies and salt. Increase the heat. Cook the vegetables for 7–10 minutes, turning them with the tongs.

3   Serve hot with lemon wedges and garnished with the fresh coriander. A sauce of thick Greek-style yogurt adds an interesting contrast, provides protein and calcium and benefits your digestion.

Spaghetti Squash with Cabbage and Nuts

Spaghetti squash is a summer squash that has earned its name from the resemblance of its cooked flesh to spaghetti pasta. It is also known as vegetable spaghetti, spaghetti marrow and noodle squash.

Serves: 4
Preparation time: 10 minutes
Cooking time: 20 minutes

1.5kg (3lb) spaghetti squash
1.5 tablespoons olive oil
2 cloves garlic, crushed
250g (8oz) green cabbage, finely shredded
75g (3oz) raw almonds or cashews
100g (3oz) crème fraiche
nutmeg, freshly grated
salt and pepper

1 Cut the pumpkin, unpeeled, into quarters, discard the seeds and cook the flesh in boiling water for about 15 minutes or until soft.

2 Heat the olive oil in a frying pan. Lightly sauté the onion and garlic for 5 minutes.

3 Add the shredded cabbage and sauté for 3 minutes or until tender.

4 Add the nuts, crème fraiche and nutmeg. Season to taste and cook until the crème fraiche melts to make a sauce. Drain the pumpkin. Scoop the flesh away from the skin. Use 2 forks to break the strands apart. Add this flesh to the rest of the mixture in the pan, heat gently for 1 minute. Serve immediately with a fresh green salad.

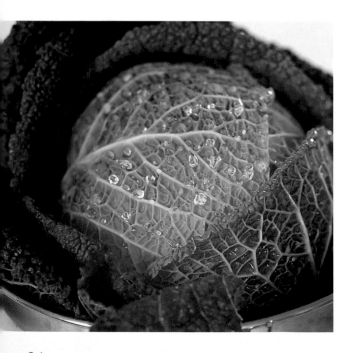

Kale and Potato Colcannon

Cabbage is a rich source of vitamins A, B and C, and a good source of iron, potassium and calcium, so this dish provides an excellent mix of nutrients and vitamins for the bones.

Serves: 4–6
Preparation time: 20 minutes
Cooking time: 20 minutes

500g (1lb) kale or green leaf cabbage, stalk removed and finely shredded
500g (1lb) potatoes, unpeeled
6 spring onions or chives, finely chopped
150ml (¼ pint) milk or natural yogurt
125g (4oz) butter
salt and pepper

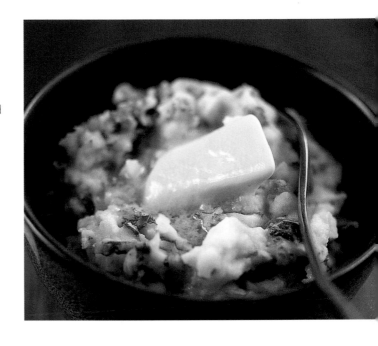

1 Place the kale or cabbage and the potatoes separately in large saucepans of boiling water and cook until tender – about 10–20 minutes for the kale or cabbage, longer for the potatoes.

2 Meanwhile, place the spring onions or chives and milk or yogurt in a small saucepan and simmer over a low heat for about 5 minutes

3 Drain the kale or cabbage. Mash with a fork so that is is ready to be added to the potato when it has been drained and mashed.

4 Drain the potatoes. Holding them in a tea towel, peel them carefully while warm and mash well with a potato masher or fork. Add the hot yogurt and spring onions, beating well to give a soft, fluffy texture.

5 Beat in the mashed kale or cabbage, season with salt and pepper, to taste, and add half the butter. The colcannon should be a speckled green colour. Heat through thoroughly then serve in warmed individual dishes or bowls. Make a well in the centre of each serving and put a knob or the remaining butter in each one. Serve immediately.

Fillet of Sole with Melon and Mint

Many of my patients say they don't like fish (low-fat) as much as meat (high-fat). When dressed up with fruit and herbs it often has more appeal.

Serves: 4
Preparation time: 20 minutes
Cooking time: 10–12 minutes

4 sole fillets, halved
2 tablespoons chopped mint
300ml (½ pint) dry white wine
1 Charentais (or other) melon, halved and deseeded
150ml (¼ pint) natural yogurt
salt and pepper
sprigs of fresh mint, to garnish

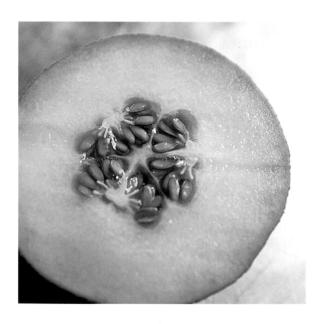

1 Season the sole fillets with salt and pepper and sprinkle with half of the chopped mint. Roll up each fish fillet and secure with wooden cocktail sticks. Place the fish rolls in a deep frying pan and sprinkle the remaining mint over them. Add the white wine. Cover the pan and poach gently for about 8 minutes, until the fish is tender.

2 Meanwhile, use a melon ball cutter to scoop the melon flesh into small balls. Cut out any remaining melon flesh attached to the skin.

3 Carefully drain the rolled fillets, place on a warm serving dish and keep warm. Remove the cocktail sticks.

4 Boil the poaching liquid with the remnants of melon flesh until well reduced and whisk until smooth. If necessary, purée in a food processor or blender. Stir in the yogurt and heat the sauce through gently. Season with salt and pepper and spoon over the cooked fish. Garnish with the melon balls and sprigs of mint. Serve with potatoes and one or more vegetable dishes.

Stir-fried Chicken with Crunchy Vegetables

I am not assuming that, in the interests of preventing osteoporosis, you will become a vegetarian, nor is there any need to do so. However, for obvious reasons the main emphasis in this recipe section has been on vegetables, soya dishes and dairy products. I am including here just a small sample of fish and meat dishes in which high-calcium dairy products or mineral-rich vegetables play a part. These ideas should stimulate you to create dishes in which vegetables are the main component, but in such a way that they complement the meat or fish you choose to serve.

Serves: 4
Preparation time: 15 minutes
Cooking time: 6–10 minutes

1 teaspoon vegetable oil
500g (1lb) chicken breasts, skinned, boned and cut into thin strips across the grain
125g (4oz) white cabbage, finely shredded
125g (4oz) bean sprouts
1 large green pepper, cored, deseeded and cut lengthways into thin strips
2 medium carrots, cut lengthways into thin strips
2 garlic cloves, crushed
freshly ground black pepper

Sauce:
2 teaspoons cornflour
4 tablespoons water
3 tablespoons soy sauce

These vegetables provide minerals, vitamins and fibre thus benefiting your bones and your digestion. As an alternative you could try other vegetables, such as green beans or broccoli.

1 Prepare the sauce. Mix the cornflour to a thin paste with the water, then stir in the soy sauce. Set aside.

2 Heat a wok until hot. Add the oil and heat over a moderate heat. Add the chicken strips, increase the heat and stir-fry for 3–4 minutes until lightly coloured on all sides. Remove from the heat and transfer the chicken to a plate with a slotted spoon.

3 Return the wok to a moderate heat until hot. Add all the vegetables and garlic and stir-fry for 2–3 minutes or until the green pepper is just beginning to soften.

4 Stir the sauce to mix it, then pour into the wok. Increase the heat to high and toss the ingredients until the sauce thickens and coats the vegetables. Add the chicken with its juices and toss for 1–2 minutes or until all the ingredients are combined. Add pepper to taste and serve at once.

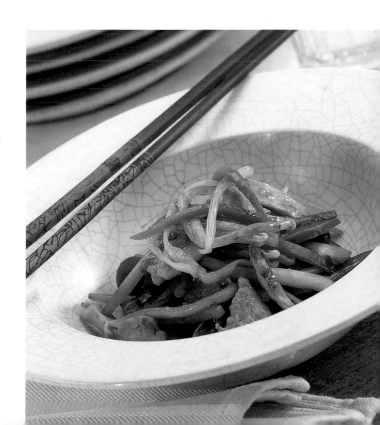

Sweet and Sour Chinese Turkey

This is an excellent example of how to combine meat with nutrient-rich vegetables to the benefit of your total health. Sharon fruit is a type of persimmon, which can be eaten like an apple. The skin is edible or, if you prefer, the fruit can be peeled.

Serves: 4
Preparation time: 15 minutes, plus marinating
Cooking time: 15–20 minutes

500g (1lb) turkey breast
2 tablespoons lemon juice
5 tablespoons orange juice
4–5 celery sticks
2 sharon fruits or firm tomatoes
8–10 radishes
½ Chinese cabbage
1 large green pepper, cored and deseeded
1 tablespoon oil
150ml (¼ pint) chicken stock
1½ teaspoons cornflour
1 tablespoon soy sauce
1 tablespoon clear honey

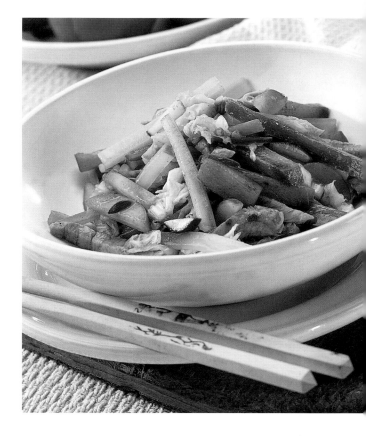

1 Cut the turkey breast into thin strips. Marinate in the lemon and orange juices for 30 minutes.

2 Cut the celery, sharon fruits or tomatoes, radishes, Chinese cabbage and green pepper into small, neat pieces.

3 Heat the oil in a large nonstick frying pan or wok. Drain the turkey and reserve the marinade. Fry the turkey in the oil until nearly tender. Add the vegetables and sharon fruits or tomatoes and heat for 2–3 minutes only.

4 Blend the chicken stock with the marinade and the cornflour. Add the soy sauce and honey. Pour this mixture over the ingredients in the pan and stir until thickened. Serve immediately, with brown rice and a large fresh vegetable salad.

Sauces

A simple dish of steamed vegetables can be made into an exciting taste sensation by the addition of well-flavoured sauces.

Dill Sauce

This is delicious with lightly steamed root vegetables.

3 tablespoons olive oil
3 tablespoons wholemeal flour
500ml (17fl oz) stock
4 tablespoons chopped fresh dill
1 tablespoon apple cider vinegar
1 tablespoon Greek yogurt
salt and pepper

Combine the oil, flour and stock and cook as for Basic 'White' Sauce (see right). Add the remaining ingredients, simmer for a further minute or two, season to taste and serve.

Beetroot Sauce

1kg (2lb) beetroot
2 tablespoons lemon juice
2 tablespoons Greek yogurt
salt and pepper

Trim the root and stems from the beetroots, being careful not to cut into the vegetable itself or it will 'bleed' and lose its distinctive colour. Boil them until tender. Leave to cool then peel.

Grate or blend the cooked beetroot. Put in a saucepan and add the lemon juice and yogurt. Stir well, heat through for a few minutes, season and serve. It makes an excellent accompaniment for meat dishes.

Basic 'White' Sauce

I long ago gave up the complex business of making a white sauce by melting butter, adding flour and slowly stirring in milk, hoping that it wouldn't go lumpy. The following method I find works perfectly well and is quick and simple to do. You can use butter instead of olive oil if you prefer, but oil is more nutritious.

1 tablespoon olive oil
300ml (½ pint) milk
1 tablespoon wholemeal flour
salt and pepper

Put the oil and milk in a saucepan. Sprinkle the flour on top. Stir or whisk briskly to blend the ingredients. Put over the heat and slowly bring to the boil, stirring from time to time as it warms and then continuously as the sauce begins to thicken. Simmer for a few minutes and season to taste.

To turn this into a cheese sauce omit the oil or butter and use 100g (3½oz) cheese to keep the sauce creamy and also add extra calcium. To provide additional piquancy add a small amount of mustard and/or freshly ground black pepper, paprika or a pinch of cayenne pepper.

The amino acids of the proteins in the milk and the flour combine well to provide a total protein intake with a high net utilization.

This sauce can be used on its own to add substance to a vegetable dish, or it can be used as the basis for a variety of other sauces, such as parsley, pepper or other herb sauces.

Lemon Grass and Tofu Nuggets with Chilli Sauce

Including generous amounts of soya beans and soya products in your diet will have special benefits for the health of your bones (see chapters 1 and 2). You can buy soya mince, fine or coarse, and use it in a range of dishes, just as you would use beef mince. Simply add it instead of the meat and use extra liquid (stock or water) to allow for the fact that it is a dried product and will take up a lot of the liquid from the recipe.

Serves: 4
Preparation time: 10 minutes
Cooking time: 10 minutes

1 bunch of spring onions
5cm (2in) piece of fresh root ginger, peeled and chopped
2 lemon grass stalks, roughly chopped
small handful of coriander
3 garlic cloves, roughly chopped
1 teaspoon honey
1 tablespoon light soy sauce
300g (10oz) tofu, drained
75g (3oz) wholemeal breadcrumbs
1 egg
oil, for shallow-frying
salt and pepper

Dipping sauce:
1 tablespoon clear honey
2 tablespoons soy sauce
1 red chilli, deseeded and sliced
2 tablespoons orange juice

1 Thinly slice 1 spring onion and set aside. Roughly chop the remainder and place in a food processor with the ginger, lemon grass, coriander and garlic. Process lightly until mixed together and chopped but still chunky. Add the honey, soy sauce, tofu, breadcrumbs, egg, salt and pepper, and process until just combined.

2 Take dessertspoonfuls of the mixture and pat into flat cakes using lightly floured hands.

3 Make the dipping sauce. Mix together the ingredients, adding the reserved sliced spring onion, in a small serving bowl.

4 Heat the oil in a large, preferably nonstick frying pan. Add half the tofu cakes and fry gently for 1–2 minutes on each side until golden. Drain on kitchen paper and keep warm while frying the remainder. Serve with the dipping sauce.

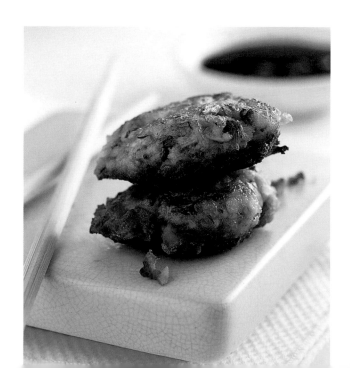

Thai-dressed Tofu Rolls

Soya tofu (bean curd) is available plain or with a variety of flavours in it. Plain tofu can be used like cottage cheese. It can be lightly sautéed and added to vegetable dishes to add protein and other benefits. The flavoured tofu lends itself to a wide range of dishes, of which the following is one example.

Serves: 4
Preparation time: 10 minutes
Cooking time: 10 minutes

1 small iceberg lettuce
275g (9oz) tofu, diced
100g (3½oz) mangetout, shredded lengthways
2 tablespoons sesame oil
2 tablespoons light soy sauce
2 tablespoons lime juice
1 tablespoon honey
1 Thai chilli, deseeded and sliced
1 garlic clove, crushed
pepper

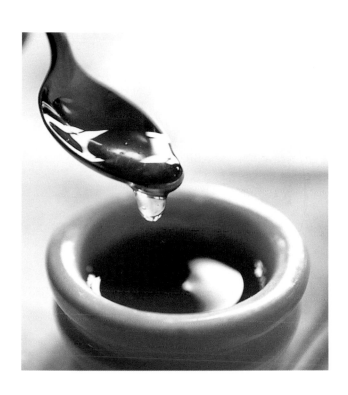

1 Remove 8 leaves from the lettuce. Fill a large, heatproof bowl with boiling water. Add the separated leaves and leave for 10 seconds. Rinse in cold water and drain thoroughly.

2 Finely shred the remaining lettuce and toss in a bowl with the tofu and mangetout.

3 Mix together the sesame oil, soy sauce, lime juice, honey, chilli, garlic and pepper and add to the tofu mixture. Toss together gently.

4 Spoon a little mixture on to the centre of each blanched lettuce leaf, then roll up. Chill until ready to serve.

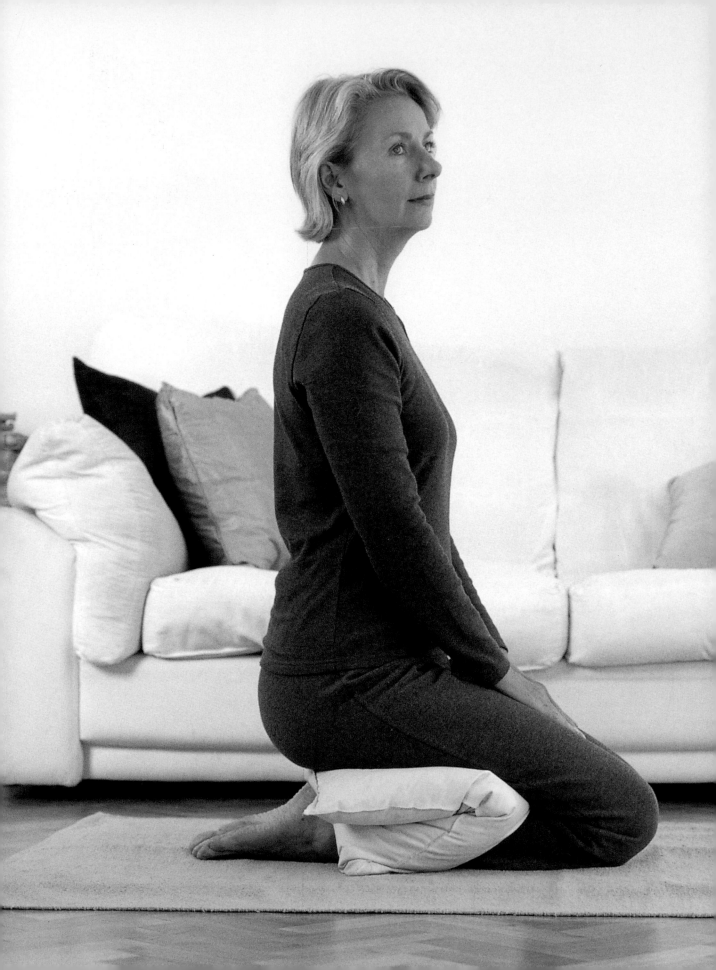

Exercises

Regular exercise accomplishes many things for your individual bones, your whole skeleton and your health in general. A full keep-fit plan would involve more radical exercises than are described here – sports, gym work, jogging and others. The following exercises have a different purpose. They are aimed at strengthening your bones and at doing so without taking a large amount of time, without needing special equipment or another person to work with and without necessitating a change of clothing. They are exercises that can be done within the normal course of your day and at any odd moment when you have time to spare.

General Fitness

If you are young and interested in the prevention of osteoporosis the exercises will be easy, and will become more so as you get fitter. If, however, you are older and your joints are stiff or your balance is poor, you should start carefully and be selective in the exercises you do. If an exercise involves jumping and this jars your bones, then either finder a softer surface on which to do it or leave it out. If in doubt, then get professional advice. In all cases, unless you are already fit and supple, start slowly and gradually make more and more demands on your body.

Build exercises into your daily life

The following simple exercises will:

- help to strengthen the different bones as they are given greater weights to carry
- maintain strength in your spine
- improve your muscle alignment, tone and balance
- increase your flexibility, stability and circulation

As a result of this there will be greater blood flow to your bones and joints, carrying oxygen and other nutrients to them, and there will be greater flow of lymph and a greater possibility of carrying toxins away from them. Some of the exercises will also increase your breathing rate and your fitness.

There are many ways to build exercises into your day. They may take a small amount of time, but the benefits are enormous, and can outweigh the effort involved. In ancient times you *had* to run or walk anywhere you wanted to go. You *had* to climb if you wanted to go up hill. Exercise was an integral part of life. It was not something you did for half an hour and ticked it off your 'to do' list. That is how it should be today. Doing small frequent amounts of exercise makes sure you keep in good shape without periods of strain or exhaustion.

Stop using lifts

There are probably many times throughout a week when you go up one or more floors in a lift. Stop. *Always* look for the stairs. Even walking downstairs is good exercise and the weight moving on to each leg as you descend helps to pump in the calcium. If necessary, start slowly. Start by walking down, then by walking up only one flight. Take the lift the rest of the way. Gradually increase both the speed at which you climb or descend and the number of flights you climb. Remember, each step you climb puts weight on some of your bones and strengthens them. Even if you live on the ground floor there must be a staircase somewhere, so walk up and down it several times a day, just for the exercise. You do not need expensive equipment when you have resources to hand that can be utilized.

Stair Jump and Skipping

Remember how much fun skipping was as a child? Well, there are serious reasons for doing this and other bone-loading exercises now.

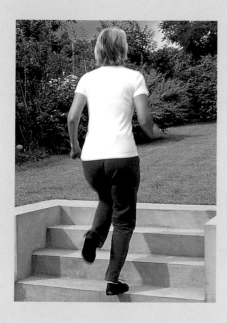

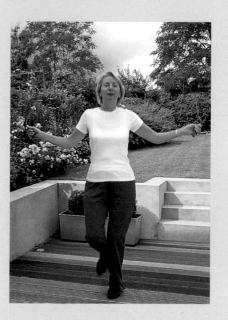

1 Once you have got used to walking up stairs again, it is time to progress. Instead of simply placing your foot on the next step and then lifting your weight on to it, do a small jump on to the upper foot. This will increase, temporarily, the weight that leg has to bear and so increase the amount of calcium entering it. As your fitness increases go up stairs a bit faster. This will increase your fitness, balance and bone strength.

1 You can skip out in the garden, in the garage or some other suitable space. If this is jarring to your knees do it on soft ground such as a lawn. Make sure there is sufficient space around you before you begin. Start slowly and gradually increase your duration and speed.

Walk up the escalators

People seem to lose the use of their legs the moment they step on to an escalator. Don't do that. Keep walking. Keep in mind that the faster you walk up the greater the number of steps you have time to climb and the greater the benefit both to your heart and your bones.

Simple steps

Do this one on your staircase. You may live in a flat without a staircase, but you can still manage to do steps. Perhaps you have a simple set of kitchen steps – one with just two steps to it to help you get things from those high cupboards. Make sure it is strong, well-balanced, stable and not likely to slip. If your balance is a little unsteady put the steps beside the wall or other firm support. Then step up, one two, down, one two. Repeat this procedure for five minutes, changing the leading step halfway through.

Simple Stretches

Use these simple stretches as 'quick-fix' exercises that can be done in any spare moments you might have.

1 Stand with your back straight and shoulders relaxed, use a chair or stick for support. Bend your left leg back and hold your ankle. Keep your thigh straight and parallel to your right leg and knees together. Hold for 10 seconds. Repeat with the other leg.

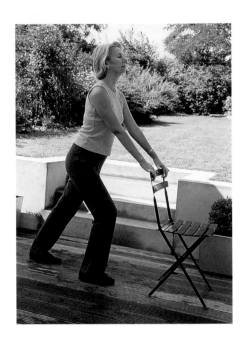

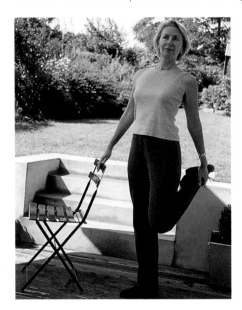

2 Use a chair for balance and stand with your legs slightly bent. Step back with your left leg, keeping it straight. Hold this for 10 seconds. Repeat with the other leg.

3 Raise your left arm above your head, keeping your hand near to a right angle, palm flat. Twist your hand, and your whole arm back and forth, almost as if you were changing a lightbulb. Do this for 30 seconds. Repeat with the other arm.

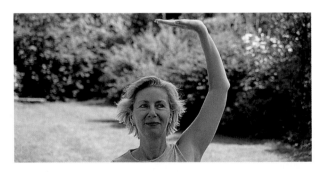

4 Cross both hands in front of your face, fingers straight. Bend and stretch each finger in turn so that they are almost touching the palm of your hand. Repeat this exercise on both hands three times.

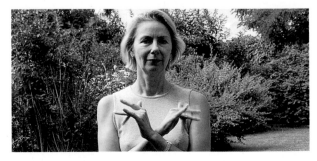

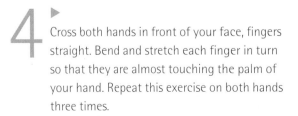

'Prayer' Stretch

These stretches are perfect for fitting into a busy schedule. Whether at home, work or just walking, you will have time to give these a go.

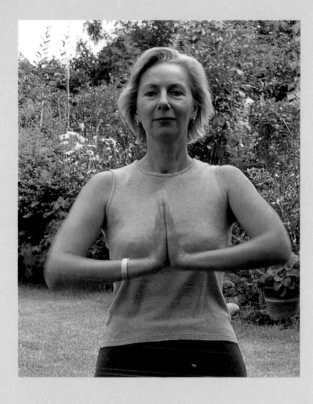

1 Hold your hands in front of you, palm to palm, as in prayer. Keep your lower arms horizontal and your elbows out to the side. Press your hands firmly together.

2 Keep your hands touching and move your fingers up and down so that they face upwards and downwards. Keep pushing your hands against each other. Repeat this 10 times.

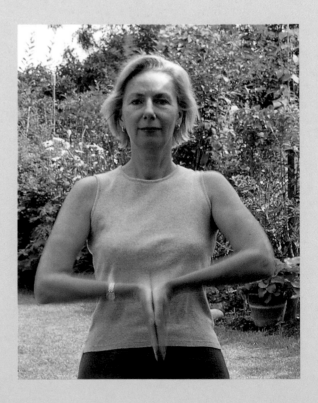

Stretching

You can of course, incorporate a full exercise session into your life. However, my suggestion here is that you build some of the following exercises into your normal daily activities. As such a warm-up session is not always necessary. If you are out of practice, a few simple stretching exercises, such as these, will help to improve your ability to be more physically active.

Rocking Feet

These are easy exercises that can be done while washing up or cooking in the kitchen, or against any waist level counter or chair.

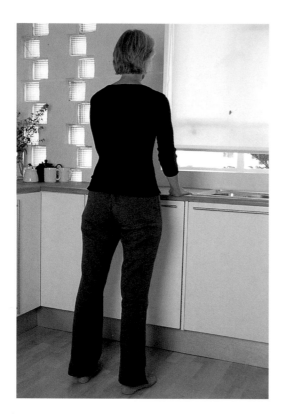

1 Stand upright using a work unit, a kitchen worktop or a chair for balance, keeping your back straight and your shoulders relaxed.

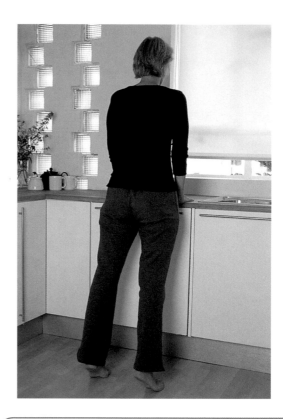

2 Raise yourself up on to your toes and hold for five seconds then release the weight back on to your heels. Repeat this 15 times.

The heel fall

Stand up while talking on the phone, this is an excellent chance to fit in some bone-benefiting exercises. Stand on your toes and let your weight fall back on your heels. Start off gently and then with increasing vigour. You will feel the pressure throughout your skeleton and this helps pump calcium into your bones.

Easy exercises

Many people say they don't have time to do exercises. This is rarely true even if you don't have time to go to a gym or do an organized exercise programme. Use the time you spend watching television, standing in queues or waiting for the kettle to boil, time that would otherwise be wasted.

Side Stretch

Keep yourself supple and improve your balance with this simple stretch that concentrates on you arms and waist.

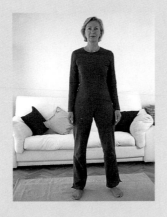

1 ◂ Stand upright with your back straight, your shoulders relaxed and your feet hip width apart.

2 ▸ Keeping your back straight and tummy held in, your right arm dropped and left hand on your hip, bend to the right. It sometimes helps to imagine that you are doing this exercise between two sheets of glass, as you should keep your back as straight as possible. Hold this position for five seconds. Stand up and repeat five times.

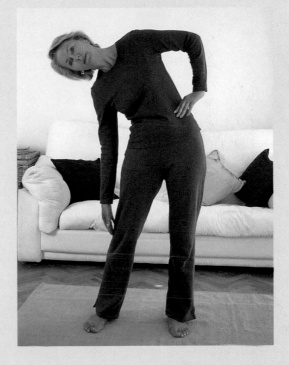

Extra benefits

For extra weight-bearing pressure, try this routine using small hand weights.

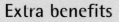

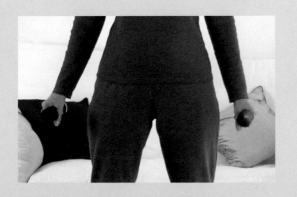

3 ▸ Repeat the exercise on the other side.

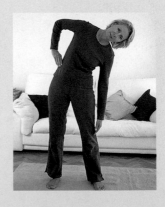

Chair Twist

While holding the telephone use the time to do this simple exercise. Put your phone on remote, or hold it in your left hand and twist to the right – then do the reverse.

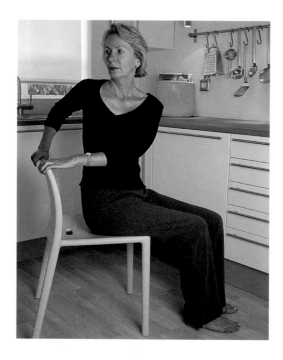

1 ◄ Sit upright in your chair, keep your buttocks firmly in place and your spine straight. Twist round to the right using your right hand to pull you round, then back.

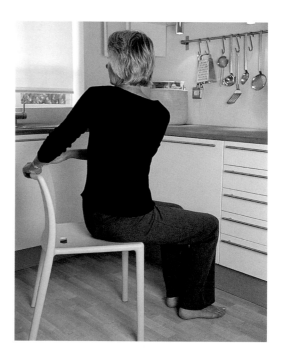

2 ▶ Change the phone to your right hand, if necessary, and swing round to the left, grasping the back of your chair with your left hand.

Run, don't walk

I recall as a child, when I ran everywhere as a matter of course, feeling sorry for adults who could only walk. It took them so much longer to get places than it took me. I swore that I would continue to run all my life, and I still do. It may only be from the house to the garden. It may only be the couple of hundred yards from my home to my office in London. However little you can do, if possible, run. Many people fear looking silly, especially in the city when they are dressed up to look smart. Yet a small amount of gentle jogging need not rearrange your hairstyle nor work you up into a lather and it will certainly be good for your health.

Chair Pick-up

*The next time you need to pick something up from floor level do the following exercises
to increase flexibility and circulation.*

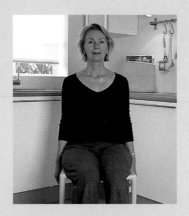

1 Start by sitting up straight, with your arms by
your side.

2 Instead of gently leaning forwards and down,
keep your spine straight and bend down
sideways to pick the item up. You will feel the
extra load on the near leg.

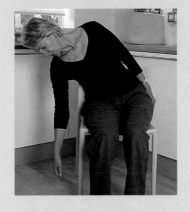

3 If you have time, extend this exercise by bringing
your other hand down to join the first. If you are
in a restaurant this may be all you do; if you are
at home, and perhaps waiting for someone else to
finish their meal, you can take the time to repeat
the exercise on the other side.

4 You can extend this exercise further by swinging
the other arm above your head.

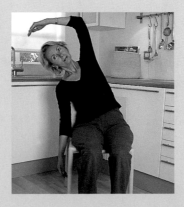

Facing Backwards

Try this exercise next time you have a spare minute when sitting in your office or your kitchen talking to someone.

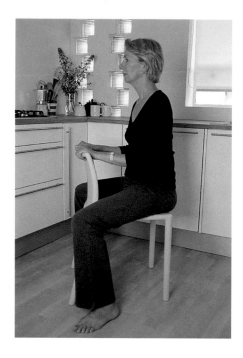

1 Turn your chair round and sit with the back of it in front of you.

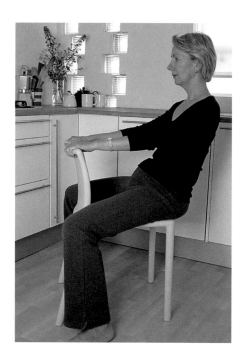

2 Hold the top of the back with both hands and lean backwards. Hold for a couple of seconds and repeat 10 times.

Pushing away from your desk

During a pause in your work put your hands flat against your desk and move as if to push yourself away, only keep your chair still and stay put. This will put beneficial pressure on your arm bones. Your desk may be beside a wall or filing cabinet. Reach your arms, one or both depending on the situation, out horizontally, put your palms against the vertical surface and push. If your desk is so placed that you can stretch your legs out in front of you and put the soles of your feet against a wall, do so, pushing against the wall while remaining in your seat, in the same position. Sit on a chair, put your hand or knuckle on the seat and push up, taking your body weight on your arms.

Work Top

Each time you stand at the sink or at the stove, make sure you put these 'spare' minutes to good use.

1 ▶ Take a step backwards, lunge forward on to one foot, letting it take your weight, and put both hands on the surface in front of you. Then lift your weight off the forward foot and let your hands and the back foot take your weight. By pressing hard with your hands you can increase the pressure on the back foot, thus pumping calcium into the bones of both arms and the back leg.

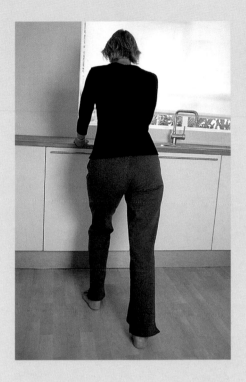

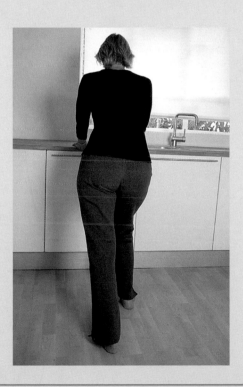

2 ◀ Repeat with the other foot. This exercise can be done at any time when you are moving around the house.

As a variation simply step back from the counter, lean on your hands and walk your legs backwards. Bend your arms so they take even more of your body weight. You are pumping calcium, all the time.

Walking jog

You may say your days of running are over, but most people can manage a walking jog. Do a 'gentle jog' whereby you make the motions of running but never actually leave the ground. You are exerting more energy, increasing your breathing rate and adding to the weight-bearing of your bones.

Feet Shift

*Do this exercise when waiting in a queue. It will increase your flexibility and encourage
circulation. If your balance is poor, hold on to a rail.*

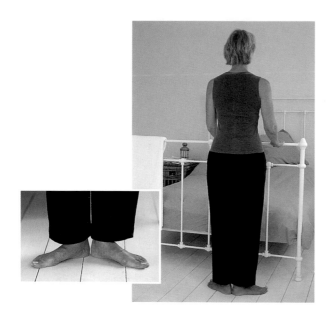

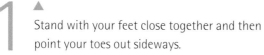

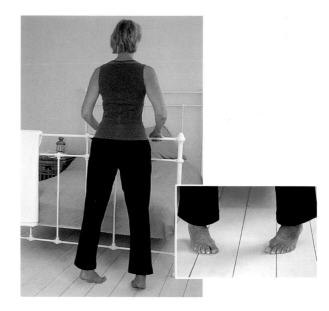

1 Stand with your feet close together and then
point your toes out sideways.

2 Transfer your weight to your toes and move your
heels out sideways.

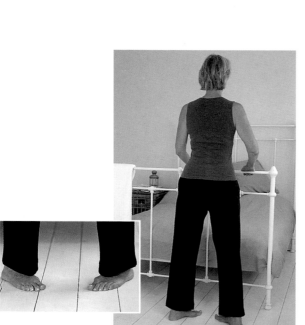

3 Bring your heels down so that the soles of your
feet are flat on the ground. Then reverse the
moves and return to your starting position.

For safety, always return to the neutral position
and do a small squatting exercise to get your
spine aligned.

Strong Arms

This exercise can be done using a strong stick or the bar of a shopping trolley while you are waiting at the checkout. Use the stick, or the back of your trolley and try to 'break it'.

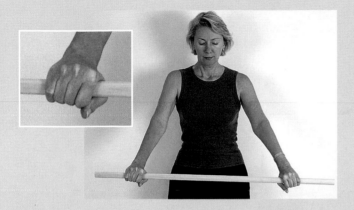

1 Hold the stick with your hands in the palms down position and try to break it as you would try to break a piece of firewood, by bringing your fists, thumbs down, in to face each other and bending both ends of the stick towards the floor (if it were flexible).

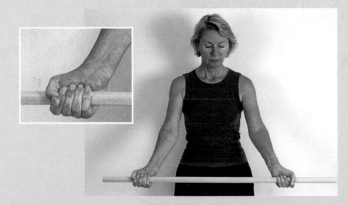

2 Then reverse the process and, with the same grip, rotate your fists so they face away from each other, thumbs up, and the ends of the stick, if it could bend, would point upwards.

In the supermarket you can do this in the same way, using the trolley rail. You can also do this exercise holding any other horizontal rail such as a banister, a fence, metal railing or the arm of a chair. If it is a long queue at the checkout you will have plenty of time to reverse the process and try to 'break' the rail in the reverse direction. Doing it in the various different ways applies load to various bones in your arms.

When you try it for yourself you will find that only a small amount of 'work' or pressure on your part will make a noticeable impact on the bones of your lower arms.

Leg stand in queues

It is almost impossible to avoid standing in queues. Put this time to good use. Instead of increasing your mental and nervous tension, welcome the time. Stand on one foot, give one leg the task of carrying your full body weight for several seconds. Bounce slightly. Swap legs and repeat. Keep repeating this until you are at the head of the queue. This will increase the total amount of load bearing on each leg alternately.

Thigh Stretch

If you have a bare wall near your television, make sure you don't waste any valuable exercising time just sitting on the sofa.

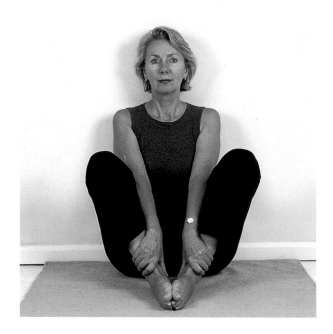

1 Sit on the floor, spine upright and back against the wall, legs out in front. Bend your knees and bring them up to your chest, grasping your ankles as you do so. Keep your arms inside your legs.

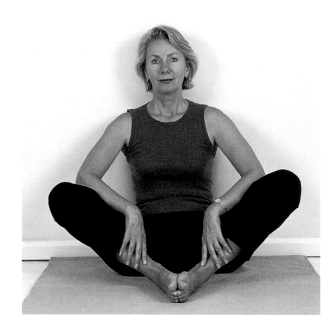

2 Use your arms to press both legs out sideways. You will feel the pull on your thighs as you do this.

Television from the floor

Do you have to sit on a chair? Why not find a place where you can sit on the floor, with your back against the wall, and watch television from there. Then you can do these exercises at the same time. While they do put weight on various bones they are also invigorating and stretching. This improves the suppleness of your joints and increases the flow of blood, oxygen and other nutrients to the bones and joints and the flow of lymph and toxins away.

Floor Arm Stretch

If you do this exercise with a small weight in your hand it will add to the amount of pressure being exerted on your bones.

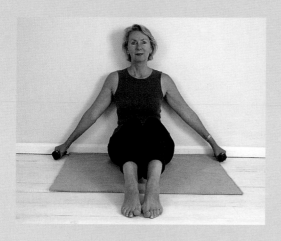

1 Sit on the floor, spine upright and back against the wall, legs straight in front of you, knees slightly bent. Keeping your spine and arms straight, stretch your arms out to each side as far as you can.

2 Lean as far as you can to one side, still keeping your spine straight. Sit up straight again and do the exercise to the other side.

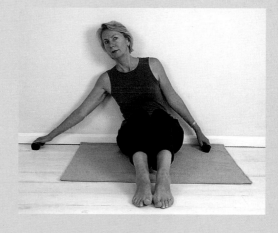

3 To extend it further, raise the arm on which you are not leaning so it is above your head and bent over. This will increase the weight on the hand that is on the floor.

109

Belt Pull

Strengthen your shoulders with this belt pull. You can use a belt, a tea towel or any handy object that can be made long and thin and pulled.

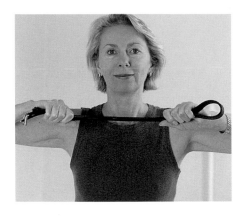

1 Grasp one end of the object in either hand and pull.

2 Lift your arms above your head while still pulling.

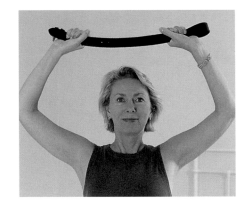

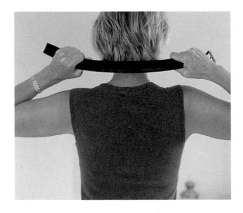

3 Lower your arms so the object is across the back of your neck and keep pulling.

4 Lower your arms again and reverse the exercise with the object behind your back.

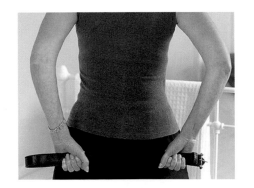

Television Pull

Next time you are watching television use the time to improve the strength of your bones in the lower arms.

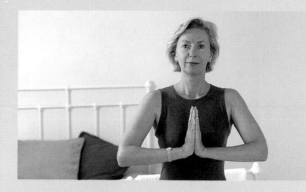

1 Hold your hands in front of you, palm to palm, as in prayer. Keep your lower arms horizontal and your elbows out to the side. Take this opportunity to pump more calcium into your bones and press your hands firmly together.

2 Then twist your arms, link your fingers together and pull firmly, as if trying to part your hands.

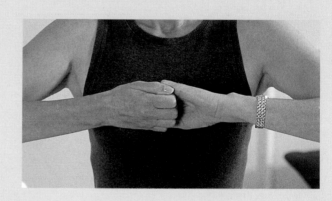

3 Slide your hands over your wrist and grab each one with the opposite hand and pull.

4 Swap positions by releasing your hold and twisting the hand that was facing your body so it faces away from you and twisting the other one in the opposite direction. Regrasp your wrists and pull again.

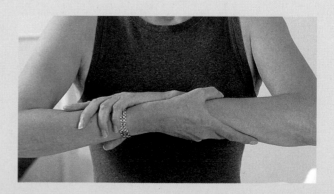

Kneel and Lunge

While the ads are on and seeing the screen is not important there are several more exercises that you can try.

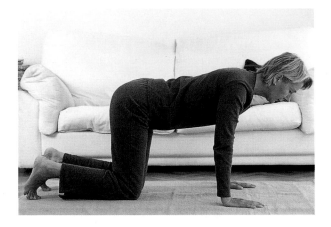

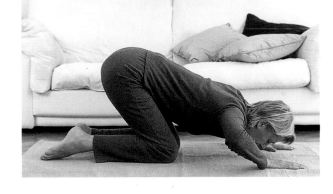

1 ▲ Kneel on all fours keeping your back straight.

2 ▲ Taking your weight on your arms, bend them until your forehead almost touches the ground. As always it is important to keep your spine straight while doing this exercise. Push yourself up with increasing vigour until you are back in the starting position. Repeat the exercise several times.

The bum lift

Sit on the floor with your hands, palm down, on either side of your buttocks and your legs straight ahead. Lift your buttocks off the ground until your body is horizontal and supported by your arms and lower legs. To extend this exercise to give greater benefit to your legs and hips gradually move your feet further from your body until your spine and legs lie in a straight line, and you are supported by your arms and heels. This is excellent for strengthening the bones of your arms and legs.

Leg Swing

This exercise will improve flexibility and circulation. If your joints are uncomfortable when leant on use a cushion for protection.

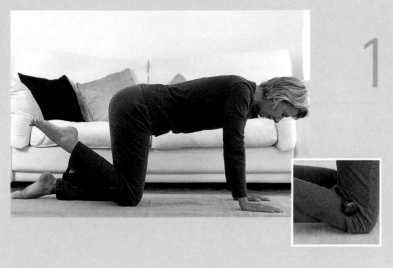

1 Kneel on all fours. You can do this exercise with or without small hand weights. If you choose to use them, place one in the bend of your right knee. Lift your lower leg slightly to keep the weight in place.

2 Lift the bent knee until it is level with your (flat) spine and your right foot is pointing up to the ceiling.

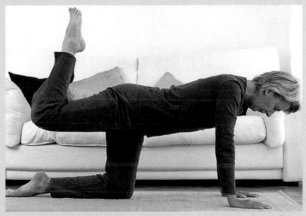

3 Swing your bent leg down and through until your knee is under your chest. Return it to the starting position and lower to the ground. Repeat the exercise using the other leg.

Kneeling Leg Lift

Remember, as shown below, to use cushions for comfort if pressure on some joints is uncomfortable.

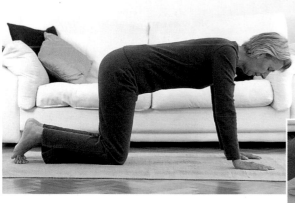

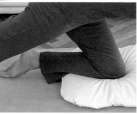

1 Kneel down on all fours. If your knees are painful, do this exercise kneeling on a cushion. Keep your face pointing down and your neck straight.

2 Straighten one leg out behind you with the toe still touching the floor and straighten it out behind you.

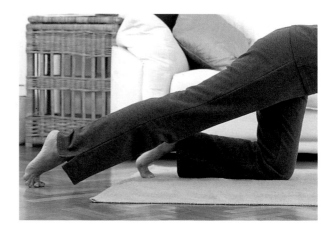

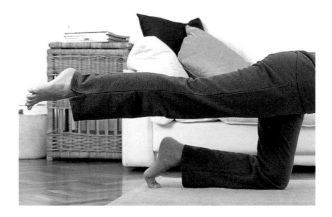

3 Gradually, lift the straightened leg up, until it is horizontal and a continuation of the spine. Hold it here for a few seconds. Lower the leg and repeat this a few times. Repeat the exercise using the other leg.

...d Walk

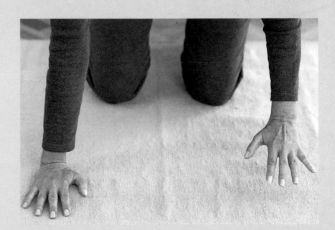

...ur hand and arm joints and bones.
...ng your head hang.

1 Kneel down on all fours, keeping your back straight.

...ing
...ine

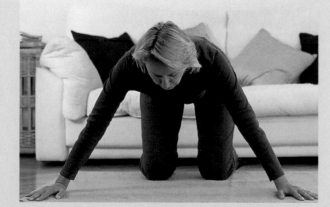

3 Now walk your hands out to the side. This will greatly increase the strength of the bones in your arms. Then walk your hands back in the reverse pattern until you are kneeling comfortably, balanced on all fours again. Repeat this a few times and then stand up. Do not be tempted to pull yourself up by a piece of furniture.

Extend the exercises on all fours by first lifting your knees off the ground and then walking your legs forward until they are underneath your body, and stand up from there. As you slowly straighten your knees, try to keep touching your toes for as long as possible; this is another useful stretch for the back of your legs.

Weight Shift

For this exercise you will need something weighty – two full litre bottles of mineral water would be ideal. Drink the water afterwards, few people drink enough.

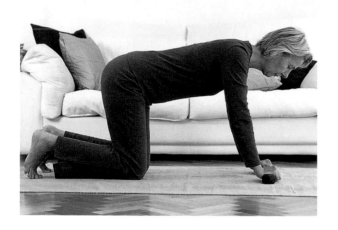

1 Kneel on all fours with one bottle or weight in each hand.

2 Lean forward keeping your spine straight and place one hand as far ahead of you as you can reach. Leave the weight at that point. Return to the normal all-fours position. Repeat the process using your other hand. Then, lean forward in a similar manner and pick up each bottle in turn and bring it back to the starting position.

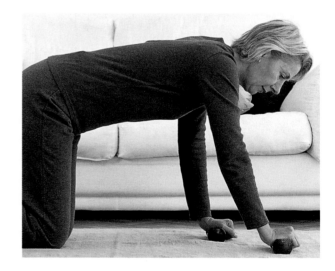

Remember

Weight-bearing exercises will increase the amount of calcium entering your bones and decrease the amount leaving, thus strengthening the bones and helping to prevent osteoporosis. Improved muscle tone is associated with increased balance and agility and so a decreased risk of bone fractures.

Relaxed Leg Lift

In case all this exercising has worn you out, here is your chance to lie down. You could even watch the television while doing this.

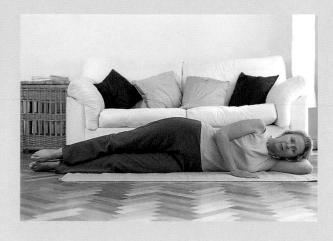

1 Lie flat on the ground, on your left side. Use your left arm to support your head.

2 Holding your right leg straight, lift it up in the air to about hip height, and hold this position for five seconds

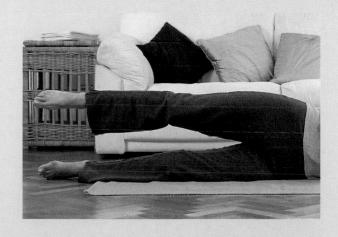

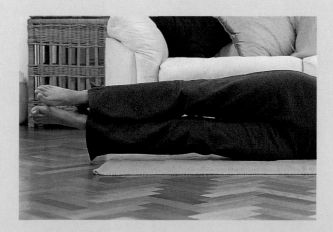

3 Lift your left leg off the ground too, until it is in mid-air, touching your right leg. Hold the position for a while, then relax and bring your legs slowly down to the ground. Turn over and lie on your right side and repeat the exercise.

If you have problems with your hips, then you may want to skip this exercise.

Hip Stretch

This is perfect for doing when watching television or while playing with the children on the floor. Ensure that you provide sufficient support for your head with your hand.

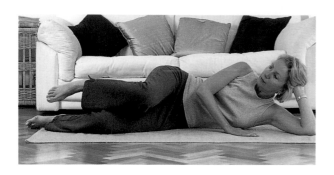

1 Lie on your left side, resting on your left elbow and using your hand to support your head. Steady yourself by putting your right hand on the floor in front of you. Your left leg should be slightly bent with your right knee pulled towards the body.

2 Extend the right leg in front of you, with the toe slightly raised from the floor. Hold this position for five seconds.

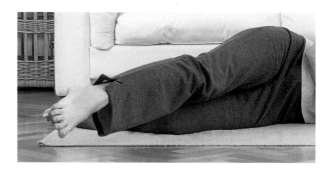

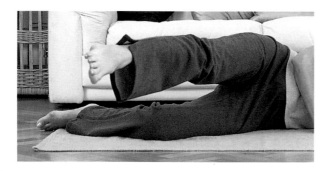

3 Lift your right leg to hip height and hold for two seconds, then lower to the floor. Repeat this exercise 15 times. Repeat the sequence 15 times on the other side.

Lazy lying-down exercises

If you are lucky enough to have a vertical bed-end that extends above the mattress level, lie on your back, work your way down the bed until your feet are flat against the bed-end, and push. This will help pump calcium into the bones of your legs. Lie on your back, lift your shoulders and prop yourself up on your elbows, then lift your buttocks off the mattress. You can also of course, do the traditional press-ups, even when confined to bed.

Leg-extender

This exercise is excellent for putting added pressure on your hip and leg joints and bones. Be careful not to push your legs too far.

1 Lie on your back with your knees bent and your arms straight out to the sides at chest level.

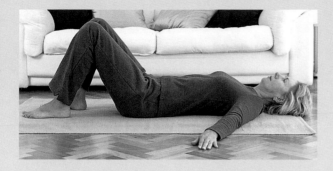

2 Drop the left knee so that your outer thigh is resting on the floor.

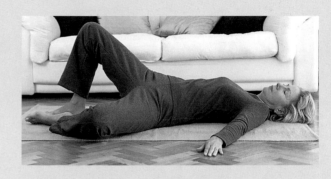

3 Straighten your right leg and lift it up and over your left leg. Hold for a few seconds.

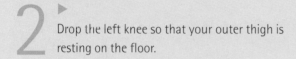

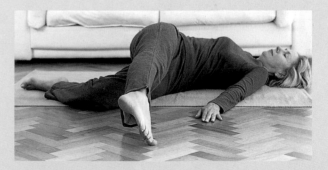

4 Push the right leg further over the left leg and drop it so that your toe is resting on the floor. Hold for a few seconds. Return your legs to the starting position. Do this several times and repeat with the other leg.

Do not force your legs if you find this uncomfortable – only push them as far as you can without strain.

Leg and Arm Lift

In this exercise you will be face down to the floor, so keep it for when there is a break in your television programme.

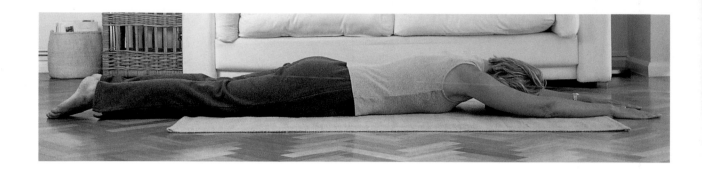

1 ▲ Lie out straight, flat on your stomach. Keep your head facing down and your forehead resting on the floor or a cushion throughout this exercise. Stretch your arms straight out ahead of you.

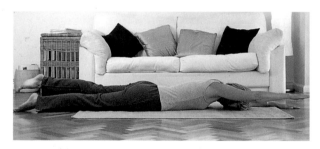

2 ◄ Raise and lower your left leg and your right arm simultaneously, keeping both of them straight. Bring them down slowly each time – do not let them fall to the ground.

3 ► Then raise your right leg and your left arm to repeat the exercise.

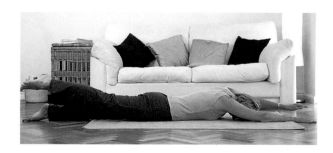

4 ◄ Finally raise both your arms and both your legs at the same time and slowly lower them to the ground.

Repeat this whole sequence several times.

Relaxation

Relaxation is an important part of exercise – just as it is vital that you exercise the bones you should also allow them to rest.

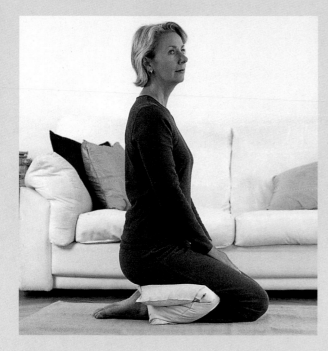

1 Assume a kneeling position on the floor. Place a cushion behind your knees and go to sit down. Your leg joints will be supported by the cushion. This is a comfortable position to relax in.

You could also use this technique when gardening or doing any work on the floor to ensure that your joints are always protected.

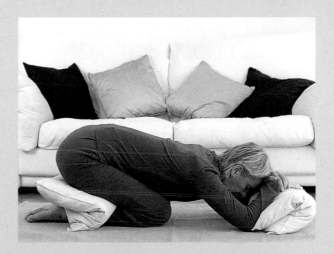

2 Keep the cushion behind your knees. Place another cushion in front of you on the floor, and lower yourself on to all fours, resting on your elbows. Your forehead and lower arms should be resting on the cushion. Hold for as long as is comfortable.

Walk

Consider how many times in the day you could walk instead of driving your car or using a bus or train. If your journey is only a short one, walk the whole way. And don't say you haven't got time, you haven't got time *not* to walk! Walking will improve your health and the state of your bones and could well increase your lifespan. It will also cut down the time you need to spend each evening on your exercise programme. Slow walking is of limited value. Striding out produces better results. Whatever you do, make the effort to go a little faster each day. Your pulse rate *should* go up. Your breathing rate *should* increase. This means you are getting aerobic exercise and improving your general fitness as well as strengthening your bones. If you can't walk the whole way, walk part of the way. Catch the bus two or three stops further down the road. Do whatever it takes to add at least some walking to your journey.

Tables

Table 1

This table shows the amount of calcium in a fixed weight of each food (3.5 oz or 100 g). However, the calorie content of 3.5 oz (100 g) of these foods varies widely. It is much easier, for instance, to eat 3.5 oz (100 g) of cucumber than the same amount of almonds.

Table 1

Food	Calcium (mg)/100g (3½oz)
Cheese, Cheddar	721
Cheese, camembert	388
Soya beans, raw	277
Almonds	266
Parsley	260
Watercress	192
Hazelnuts	188
Brazil nuts	176
Milk, goats'	134
Broccoli	123
Yogurt, natural	121
Milk, cows'	119
Beet greens	119
Sunflower seeds	116
Buckwheat	114
Spinach	101
Walnuts	94
Cream	82
Okra	81
Macadamia nuts	70
Cheese, cottage	60
Peanuts	58
Swedes	58
Eggs, hens'	56
Leeks	56
Oats	55
Parsnip	54
Red lentils, raw	51
Swiss chard	51
Kohlrabi	50
Turnips	49
Globe artichokes	48
Beans, green	48
Celery	48
Cabbage, white	47
Cabbage, Chinese	46

Table 2

Food	Calcium (mg)/100 cals (418 Kjoules)
Watercress	914
Beet greens	496
Parsley	473
Spinach	404
Broccoli	351
Cabbage, Chinese	329
Celery	267
Marrows	250
Okra	238
Yogurt, natural	198
Milk, goats'	194
Lettuce	188
Cucumber	186
Cabbage, white	181
Cheese, Cheddar	179
Milk, cows'	178
Radish	176
Kohlrabi	172
Swiss chard	170
Turnips	169
Courgette	165
Swedes	161
Beans, green	150
Cabbage, red	135
Leeks	130
Cheese, camembert	129
Globe artichokes	120
Carrots	111
Asparagus	105
Onions	89
Oranges	85
Pumpkin	81
Cauliflower	81
Parsnip	77
Tomatoes	68
Soya beans, raw	67

Table 3

Food	Magnesium (mg)/100g (3½oz)
Broccoli	388
Sunflower seeds	354
Almonds	296
Hazelnuts	285
Soya beans, raw	280
Buckwheat	229
Brazil nuts	225
Peanuts	180
Walnuts	169
Wheat	160
Oats	144
Macadamia nuts	116
Cabbage, white	113
Red lentils, raw	107
Beet greens	106
Spinach	88
Okra	57
Kidney beans, cooked	45
Broad beans	38
Kohlrabi	37
Dates	35
Beans, green	32
Parsnip	32
Sweet potatoes	31
Watercress	30
Brussels sprouts	29
Brown rice, cooked	29
Bananas	29
Salmon	29
Cheese, Cheddar	28
Cod	28
Beetroot	25
Cream	25
Cauliflower	24
Leeks	23
Carrots	23

Table 4

Food	Magnesium (mg)/100 cals (418 Kjoules)
Broccoli	1109
Beet greens	442
Cabbage, white	435
Spinach	352
Okra	168
Watercress	143
Kohlrabi	128
Celery	122
Beans, green	100
Cabbage, Chinese	100
Asparagus	95
Cauliflower	92
Radish	88
Swiss chard	81
Cucumber	79
Sweet peppers	69
Turnips	69
Buckwheat	68
Soya beans, raw	67
Lettuce	65
Eggplant	64
Carrots	64
Tomatoes	64
Beetroot	63
Sunflower seeds	62
Brussels sprouts	59
Mushrooms	59
Leeks	53
Almonds	50
Wheat	48
Pumpkin	46
Parsnip	46
Hazelnuts	45
Swedes	42
Oats	37
Raspberries	37

Table 2

This table shows the amount of calcium in 100 calories (418 Kilojoules) of each food. This is more useful as you eat a similar amount of calories of food each day, not a similar weight of food. The most nutrient dense food is the food with the most nutrient per calorie.

Tables 3 and 4

These two tables present the same information as found in tables 1 and 2, but for the nutrient magnesium.

Food	Value
Cabbage, red	42
Oranges	40
Carrots	40
Shallots	37
Wheat	36
Figs	35
Dates	32
Sweet potatoes	32
Milk, human	32
Brussels sprouts	32
Lettuce	32
Onions	31
Radishes	30
Kidney beans, cook	28
Courgette	28
Jerusalem artichokes	26
Beetroot	26
Cucumber	26
Broad beans	22
Raspberries	22
Asparagus	22
Pumpkin	21
Cauliflower	21
Chicken	16
Tomatoes	15
Marrow	15
Apricots	14
Strawberries	14
Bamboo shoots	13
Aubergines	12
Brown rice, cooked	11
Grapes	11
Cod	10
Sweet peppers	10
Lamb	10
Pork chop	9
Salmon	8
Beef	8
Potato	7
Apples	7
Mushrooms	7
Bananas	6

Food	Value
Brussels sprouts	65
Beetroot	65
Cheese, cottage	58
Shallots	51
Aubergines	48
Figs	47
Strawberries	47
Milk, human	46
Almonds	45
Raspberries	45
Sweet peppers	38
Jerusalem artichokes	38
Eggs, hens'	35
Buckwheat	34
Mushrooms	32
Hazelnuts	30
Apricots	29
Sweet potatoes	28
Brazil nuts	27
Cream	23
Kidney beans, cooked	22
Broad beans	22
Sunflower seeds	21
Grapes	16
Red lentils, raw	15
Walnuts	15
Oats	14
Cod	14
Apples	13
Dates	12
Bamboo shoots	12
Wheat	11
Peanuts	11
Macadamia nuts	10
Potatoes	10
Brown rice, cooked	9
Chicken	8
Bananas	7
Lamb	7
Salmon	5
Pork chop	3
Beef	2

Food	Value
Celery	22
Potato	22
Turnips	20
Cheese, camembert	20
Asparagus	20
Raspberries	18
Sweet peppers	18
Figs	17
Aubergines	16
Beef	16
Radish	15
Swedes	15
Pork chop	15
Parsley	14
Cabbage, Chinese	14
Milk, goats'	14
Tomatoes	14
Milk, cows'	13
Mushrooms	13
Lamb	13
Yogurt, natural	12
Onions	12
Pumpkin	12
Eggs, hens'	12
Lettuce	11
Cucumber	11
Jerusalem artichokes	11
Oranges	10
Strawberries	10
Apricots	8
Grapes	6
Cheese, cottage	5
Apples	5
Milk, human	3
Bamboo shoots	3
Marrows	0
Swiss chard	0
Courgettes	0
Cabbage, red	0
Globe artichokes	0
Shallots	0
Chicken	0

Food	Value
Broad beans	36
Cod	36
Kidney beans, cooked	35
Brazil nuts	34
Onions	34
Strawberries	33
Peanuts	32
Red lentils, raw	32
Bananas	32
Potatoes	32
Sweet potatoes	29
Walnuts	27
Parsley	26
Brown rice, cooked	25
Figs	24
Oranges	23
Milk, goats'	21
Yogurt, natural	20
Milk, cows'	20
Apricots	19
Macadamia nuts	17
Jerusalem artichokes	17
Salmon	16
Dates	13
Apples	13
Grapes	8
Eggs, hens'	8
Lamb	8
Cheese, Cheddar	7
Cream	7
Cheese, camembert	7
Pork chop	7
Cheese, cottage	6
Beef	5
Milk, human	5
Bamboo shoots	4
Marrows	3
Courgettes	0
Cabbage, red	0
Globe artichokes	0
Shallots	0
Chicken	0

Tables

Table 5

The information here presents the list of foods that are covered in all the tables and their calorie content per 3.5 oz (100 g).

Table 5

Food	Calories (Kjoules)/100g (3½oz)
Almonds	589 (2,465)
Apples	59 (247)
Apricots	48 (201)
Asparagus	21 (88)
Aubergine	25 (105)
Bamboo shoots	113 (473)
Bananas	92 (385)
Beans, green	32 (134)
Beef	353 (1,477)
Beet greens	24 (100)
Beetroot	40 (167)
Brazil nuts	656 (2,745)
Broad beans	105 (439)
Broccoli	35 (146)
Brown rice, cooked	120 (502)
Brussels sprouts	49 (205)
Buckwheat	335 (1,402)
Cabbage, Chinese	14 (59)
Cabbage, red	31 (130)
Cabbage, white	26 (109)
Carrots	36 (151)
Cauliflower	26 (109)
Celery	18 (75)
Cheese, Camembert	300 (1,256)
Cheese, Cheddar	403 (1,687)
Cheese, cottage	103 (431)
Chicken	199 (833)
Cod	78 (326)
Courgettes	17 (71)
Cream	364 (1,523)
Cucumber	14 (59)
Dates	275 (1,151)
Eggs, hens'	158 (661)
Figs	74 (310)
Globe artichokes	40 (167)
Grapes	71 (297)

Table 6

Food	Magnesium: Calcium
Bananas	4.83:1
Wheat	4.44:1
Salmon	3.63:1
Broccoli	3.15:1
Potatoes	3.14:1
Peanuts	3.10:1
Sunflower seeds	3.05:1
Cod	2.80:1
Brown rice, cooked	2.64:1
Oats	2.62:1
Cabbage, white	2.40:1
Beef	2.29:1
Red lentils, raw	2.10:1
Buckwheat	2.01:1
Pork chop	1.88:1
Mushrooms	1.86:1
Sweet peppers	1.80:1
Walnuts	1.80:1
Broad beans	1.73:1
Macadamia nuts	1.66:1
Kidney beans, cook	1.61:1
Hazelnuts	1.52:1
Lamb	1.44:1
Aubergines	1.33:1
Brazil nuts	1.28:1
Cauliflower	1.14:1
Almonds	1.11:1
Dates	1.09:1
Soya beans, raw	1.01:1
Sweet potatoes	0.97:1
Beetroot	0.96:1
Tomatoes	0.93:1
Asparagus	0.91:1
Brussels sprouts	0.91:1
Beet greens	0.89:1
Spinach	0.87:1

Table 7

Food	Calcium: Phosphorus
Watercress	3.69:1
Parsley	3.61:1
Beet greens	2.98:1
Oranges	2.86:1
Figs	2.50:1
Milk, human	2.29:1
Raspberries	1.83:1
Spinach	1.74:1
Broccoli	1.60:1
Cabbage, white	1.57:1
Turnips	1.53:1
Swedes	1.49:1
Celery	1.41:1
Cheese, Cheddar	1.41:1
Cream	1.37:1
Okra	1.29:1
Milk cows'	1.28:1
Yogurt, natural	1.27:1
Marrows	1.25:1
Milk, goats'	1.21:1
Cabbage, red	1.20:1
Cabbage, Chinese	1.15:1
Lettuce	1.14:1
Cheese, camembert	1.12:1
Carrots	1.11:1
Swiss chard	1.11:1
Cucumber	1.08:1
Leeks	1.06:1
Beans, green	1.04:1
Apples	1.00:1
Kohlrabi	0.98:1
Radish	0.97:1
Courgettes	0.91:1
Grapes	0.85:1
Dates	0.80:1
Onions	0.78:1

Table 8

Food	Phosphorus: Calcium
Salmon	23.25:1
Cod	19.40:1
Pork chop	19.00:1
Beef	17.57:1
Chicken	16.75:1
Mushrooms	16.57:1
Lamb	14.44:1
Wheat	10.64:1
Red lentils, raw	8.90:1
Brown rice, cooked	8.18:1
Potatoes	7.57:1
Oats	6.75:1
Peanuts	6.60:1
Sunflower seeds	6.08:1
Kidney beans, cooked	5.07:1
Broadbeans	4.32:1
Bamboo shoots	3.85:1
Brazil nuts	3.41:1
Walnuts	3.37:1
Bananas	3.32:1
Eggs, hens'	3.21:1
Cauliflower	3.05:1
Sweet peppers	3.00:1
Jerusalem artichokes	3.00:1
Soya beans, raw	2.54:1
Buckwheat	2.47:1
Brussels sprouts	2.47:1
Asparagus	2.36:1
Cheese, cottage	2.20:1
Aubergines	2.17:1
Tomatoes	2.13:1
Pumpkin	2.10:1
Almonds	1.95:1
Macadamia nuts	1.94:1
Globe artichokes	1.83:1
Hazelnuts	1.66:1

Table 6

The figures in this column have been calculated by dividing the amount of magnesium per 100 cals (418 kjoules) by the amount of calcium per 100 cals (418 kjoules). This means that broccoli, for example, has 3.15 mg of magnesium to every 1 mg of calcium. A magnesium to calcium ratio of between 0.5:1 and 3:1 is generally considered to be ideal.

Tables 7 and 8

Table 7: A diet with approximately equal amounts of calcium and phosphorus, a ratio of around 1:1, is desirable. Few foods contain much more calcium than phosphorus.

Table 8: Foods with a very high phosphorus to calcium ratio (23.25:1 for salmon, for example) are very common.

Food	Calories (kjoules)
Hazelnuts	632 (2,645)
Jerusalem artichokes	68 (285)
Kidney beans, cooked	127 (531)
Kohlrabi	29 (121)
Lamb	186 (778)
Leeks	43 (180)
Lettuce	17 (71)
Macadamia nuts	702 (2,938)
Marrows	6 (25)
Milk, goats'	69 (289)
Milk, human	70 (293)
Milk, cows'	67 (280)
Mushrooms	22 (92)
Oats	388 (1,624)
Okra	34 (142)
Onions	35 (146)
Oranges	47 (197)
Parsley	55 (230)
Parsnip	70 (293)
Peanuts	567 (2,373)
Pork chop	234 (979)
Potatoes	76 (318)
Pumpkin	26 (109)
Radish	17 (71)
Raspberries	49 (205)
Red lentils, raw	338 (1,415)
Salmon	217 (908)
Shallots	72 (301)
Soya beans, raw	416 (1,741)
Spinach	25 (105)
Strawberries	30 (126)
Sunflower seeds	570 (2,385)
Swedes	36 (151)
Sweet peppers	26 (109)
Sweet potatoes	114 (477)
Swiss chard	30 (126)
Tomatoes	22 (92)
Turnips	29 (121)
Walnuts	642 (2,687)
Watercress	21 (88)
Wheat	330 (1,381)
Yogurt, natural	61 (255)

Food	Ratio
Raspberries	0.82:1
Kohlrabi	0.74:1
Strawberries	0.71:1
Apples	0.71:1
Okra	0.70:1
Beans, green	0.67:1
Parsnip	0.59:1
Carrots	0.58:1
Pumpkin	0.57:1
Apricots	0.57:1
Grapes	0.55:1
Radish	0.50:1
Figs	0.49:1
Swiss chard	0.48:1
Celery	0.46:1
Cucumber	0.42:1
Jerusalem artichokes	0.42:1
Leeks	0.41:1
Turnips	0.41:1
Onions	0.39:1
Lettuce	0.34:1
Cream	0.30:1
Cabbage, Chinese	0.30:1
Swedes	0.26:1
Oranges	0.25:1
Bamboo shoots	0.23:1
Eggs, hens'	0.21:1
Watercress	0.16:1
Milk, cows'	0.11:1
Milk, goats'	0.10:1
Yogurt, natural	0.10:1
Milk, human	0.09:1
Cheese, cottage	0.08:1
Parsley	0.05:1
Cheese, camembert	0.05:1
Cheese, Cheddar	0.04:1
Courgettes	*
Cabbage, red	*
Globe artichokes	*
Shallots	*
Marrows	*
Chicken	*

Food	Ratio
Strawberries	0.74:1
Apricots	0.74:1
Beetroot	0.68:1
Parsnip	0.68:1
Sweet potatoes	0.68:1
Shallots	0.62:1
Hazelnuts	0.60:1
Globe artichokes	0.55:1
Macadamia nuts	0.51:1
Almonds	0.51:1
Pumpkin	0.48:1
Tomatoes	0.47:1
Aubergines	0.46:1
Cheese, cottage	0.45:1
Asparagus	0.42:1
Brussels sprouts	0.41:1
Buckwheat	0.40:1
Scya beans, raw	0.39:1
Sweet peppers	0.33:1
Jerusalem artichokes	0.33:1
Cauliflower	0.33:1
Eggs, hens'	0.31:1
Bananas	0.30:1
Walnuts	0.30:1
Brazil nuts	0.29:1
Bamboo shoots	0.26:1
Broad bears	0.23:1
Kidney beans, cooked	0.20:1
Sunflower seeds	0.16:1
Peanuts	0.15:1
Oats	0.15:1
Potato	0.13:1
Brown rice cooked	0.12:1
Red lentils, raw	0.11:1
Wheat	0.09:1
Lamb	0.07:1
Mushrooms	0.06:1
Chicken	0.06:1
Beef	0.06:1
Pork chop	0.05:1
Cod	0.05:1
Salmon	0.04:1

Food	Ratio
Shallots	1.62:1
Sweet potatoes	1.47:1
Parsnip	1.46:1
Beetroot	1.46:1
Strawberries	1.36:1
Apricots	1.36:1
Onions	1.29:1
Dates	1.25:1
Grapes	1.18:1
Courgettes	1.04:1
Radish	1.03:1
Kohlrabi	1.02:1
Apples	1.00:1
Beans, green	0.96:1
Leeks	0.95:1
Cucumber	0.92:1
Swiss chard	0.90:1
Carrots	0.90:1
Cheese, camembert	0.89:1
Lettuce	0.88:1
Cabbage, Chinese	0.87:1
Cabbage, red	0.83:1
Milk, goats'	0.83:1
Marrows	0.80:1
Yogurt, natural	0.79:1
Milk, cows'	0.78:1
Okra	0.78:1
Cream	0.73:1
Cheese, Cheddar	0.71:1
Celery	0.71:1
Swedes	0.67:1
Turnips	0.65:1
Cabbage, white	0.64:1
Broccoli	0.63:1
Spinach	0.57:1
Raspberries	0.55:1
Milk, human	0.44:1
Figs	0.40:1
Oranges	0.35:1
Beet greens	0.34:1
Parsley	0.28:1
Watercress	0.27:1

* no magnesium content

Index

Picture credits

Getty Images/Image Bank 5 left, 34, 42-43, /Stone 30, 32.
Octopus Publishing Group Limited/Gerard Brown 27 top left,
/Jeremy Hopley 22, 60, /Sandra Lane 27 bottom right, 50, 73, 84,
/Gary Latham 41, 68, /David Loftus 58, /Peter Myers 33, /William
Reavell 1 right, 21, 36, 48, 54, 75, 78, 79, 86, 90, 91, /Niki Sianni 1
left, 3 centre, 7, 15, 25, 44, 63, 92-93, 94 left, 95 right, 96 top left,
96 top right, 96 centre right, 96 bottom right, 97 top left, 97 bottom
right, 98 left, 98 right, 99 top left, 99 centre right, 99 bottom right,
99 bottom left, 100 left, 100 right, 101 top left, 101 centre left, 101
centre right, 101 bottom right, 102 left, 102 right, 103 left, 103 right,
104 top left, 104 top right, 104 bottom left, 104 bottom centre, 104
top centre right, 104 top centre left, 105 top centre, 105 top left,
105 bottom left, 105 bottom centre, 106 top left, 106 centre right,
106 bottom left, 107 top centre, 107 top left, 107 top right, 107
bottom right, 107 bottom left, 107 bottom centre, 108 left, 108 right,
109 top left, 109 centre right, 109 bottom left, 110 top left, 110
centre left, 110 centre right, 110 bottom right, 111 top left, 111 centre
left, 111 centre right, 111 bottom right, 112 left, 112 right, 113 top
centre, 113 top left, 113 centre right, 113 bottom left, 114 top centre,
114 top left, 114 centre right, 114 bottom left, 115 top left, 115
centre right, 115 bottom left, 116 top left, 116 centre right, 117 top
left, 117 centre right, 117 bottom left, 118 top left, 118 centre right,
118 bottom left, 119 top left, 119 centre left, 119 centre right, 119
bottom right, 120 top left, 120 centre left, 120 centre right, 120
bottom right, 121 top left, 121 centre right, /Simon Smith 5 right, 57
bottom right, 81, 82, 83, 87, 88, /Ian Wallace 3 left, 35, 39, 40, 59,
62, 64, 66, 69, 74 /Philip Webb 47, 70, 85, /Mark Winwood 3 right, 6,
/William Lingwood 57 top left, /Jacqui Wornell 53.
Photodisc 28.
Science Photo Library 8-9, /Martyn F. Chillmaid 61, /Alfred Pasieka
16, /Cristina Pedrazzini 31, /Princess Margaret Rose Orthopaedic
Hospital 12, /Sheila Terry 23.

Xandria Williams

Other books currently available by Xandria Williams:

Choosing Health Intentionally
Choosing Weight Intentionally
The Four Temperaments
Beating the Blues
You're Not Alone
Living with Allergies
Fatigue – The Secrets of Getting Your Energy Back
Overcoming Candida
Liver Detox Plan
From Stress to Success

Supplements by Xandria Williams:

'Liver detox' – contains the nutrients and herbs recommended in
Liver Detox Plan
'Destress' – a combination of the nutrients and herbs recommended
in From *Stress to Success*

Ordering:

The books can be ordered from good book shops or from Xandria
Williams. The supplements can be ordered from Nutri Imports on
0-800-212-742 or from Xandria Williams (contact details on page 4).
www.xandriawilliams.com

Executive Editor Anna Southgate
Editor Abi Rowsell
Design Manager Tokiko Morishima
Production Controller Jo Sim
Picture Researcher Zoë Holterman

Special Photography Nikki Sianni
Model Helga Du Sauzay